HAPPY MIND,
HAPPY LIFE

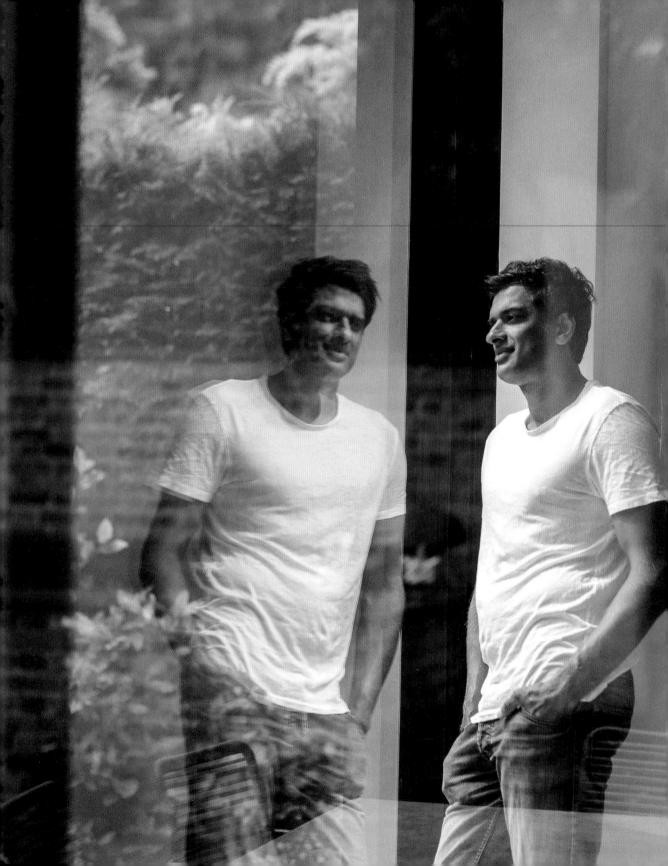

HAPPY MIND, HAPPY LIFE

10 Simple Ways to Feel Great Every Day

DR RANGAN CHATTERJEE

Photography by Chris Terry

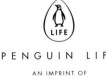

PENGUIN LIFE

AN IMPRINT OF

PENGUIN BOOKS

PENGUIN LIFE

UK | USA | Canada | Ireland | Australia
India | New Zealand | South Africa

Penguin Life is part of the Penguin Random House group of companies
whose addresses can be found at global.penguinrandomhouse.com.

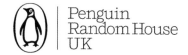

First published 2022
001

Colour reproduction by Altaimage Ltd
Printed in Italy by Printer Trento S.r.l.

The authorized representative in the EEA is Penguin Random House Ireland,
Morrison Chambers, 32 Nassau Street, Dublin D02 YH68

A CIP catalogue record for this book is available from the British Library

ISBN: 978–0–241–39785–5

www.greenpenguin.co.uk

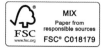

MIX
Paper from
responsible sources
FSC® C018179

Penguin Random House is committed to a
sustainable future for our business, our readers
and our planet. This book is made from Forest
Stewardship Council® certified paper.

For Vidhaata,
Jainam and Anoushka

CONTENTS

INTRODUCTION

I'd like you to take a few seconds to recall a moment from childhood when you felt truly happy. Imagine it fully: picture the colours, smell the smells, feel the weather on your cheeks and the ground beneath your feet. Where were you? Outside, perhaps? Barefoot on a sunny day, playing with a gang of friends, lost in the sheer pleasure of a game. You weren't anxious about the future. You weren't fretting about the past. You were living entirely in the moment, filled to the brim with the simple joy of being alive. So, what happened? Why aren't you that person any longer? Where did all that happiness go?

I know that life can feel tough at times. Many of us feel overwhelmed and close to burnout, with too many things to do and not enough time to do them. But whether you are struggling to keep your head above water or you simply want to feel a little bit happier than you currently are, you have come to the right place. This book will help you improve your health and your happiness. And the good news is that it's a lot easier than you think.

HAPPINESS IS MORE
THAN IT SEEMS

I've been a practising doctor for over twenty years. During that time, I've always been driven by a desire to fully understand, why is this patient sitting in front of me? What's happened in their life that's led them to my door? I've written in my previous books about the critically important role our modern lifestyle plays in the vast majority of cases I see. When people arrive with a set of physical symptoms and I do a bit of investigating, I usually find the upstream causes of their issues are to do with their food choices, a lack of regular movement, poor-quality sleep or unmanaged stress. It's amazing how often small tweaks in someone's lifestyle can have massively beneficial downstream effects on their overall health. For example, helping someone sleep better and teaching them a simple one-minute breathing exercise can have a transformative impact on someone struggling with anxiety. And someone who struggles with debilitating gut symptoms can often feel significantly better by learning how to lower their stress levels and making a few changes to their diet.

But a few years ago I began to wonder if there could be a factor that lies even further upstream than a healthy lifestyle. Could there actually be something that's even more important than food, rest and exercise? This idea kept niggling away at me. I asked myself, what about the people who are making all the right lifestyle choices and *still* find themselves having problems with their health? What's going on with them? Is there something they tend to have in common? And what about those patients who always seem to be walking a tightrope – who manage to make helpful lifestyle changes for a few weeks, or even a few months, but then revert back to their previous unhelpful behaviours? And what is it that enables some people to effortlessly make healthy choices whereas others seem to find it painstakingly hard?

Most people would tell you this all comes down to motivation and willpower. Popular belief has it that if we want to get healthy badly enough, we'll find the inner strength to do so. Success comes from mental strength, and failure comes from mental weakness. I think this is wrong. Our day-to-day habits are *not* a reflection of our strength or weakness of mind. They're a reflection of how we feel about ourselves and the world around us.

This is how it works. When we think negative thoughts and allow the actions of others to influence the way that we feel, we bring stress into our body. And stress is implicated in about 90 per cent of what a doctor like me sees on any given day. But when we feel calm, content and in control of our lives, the opposite is true: we become healthier. Time and time again I've seen this to be true: when we feel truly and deeply happy *in* our lives and *with* our lives, the knock-on consequences for our health are profound.

UPSTREAM

• How you feel about yourself and the world
• Your thoughts and emotions
• Your mental health and wellbeing

• Your day-to-day behaviours
• Your approach to food, movement, sleep and rest

Your physical health

DOWNSTREAM

HAPPINESS EQUALS HEALTHY

This link between happiness and health has been confirmed by many amazing researchers. When I spoke with the brilliant psychologist Professor Laurie Santos from Yale University she told me, 'If you look at people's happiness, you see effects on their health and longevity.' In one study, scientists brought people into the lab and measured their general positivity levels. They then shot rhinoviruses up their nostrils, which cause the common cold. Everyone in the study was exposed to the virus. The question was, who would get sick, the happy people or the unhappy ones? 'What they found was that three times the number of people got sick in the not-so-positive mood category,' Professor Santos told me.

Part of the reason happiness impacts our health so much is that, if you're feeling good about your life, you're more likely to exercise, socialize and avoid comfort foods. That's pretty obvious. But happiness goes much deeper than this. Incredibly, it's been found that, even when these kinds of lifestyle factors are accounted for, happier people still live longer. One study looked at nuns, who all ate the same diet and took similar amounts of exercise to each other. When these nuns entered service and took their Holy Orders, they all wrote an autobiographical essay. These essays were rated by psychologists, who assessed them for the amount of positive emotion they showed. The researchers then separated them into four groups, with the happiest at the top. Of that happiest quarter, 90 per cent of the nuns were still alive at the age of eighty-five. In the unhappiest quarter, just 34 per cent were still alive.

Extraordinary findings like these show us how incredibly beneficial happiness can be to our health. They confirm my own decades of experience as a doctor. So many of my patients are rushing around, struggling to find time to do simple activities like going for a walk. They're not getting enough quality sleep and are constantly feeling a background state of overwhelm. We somehow think we can live this way for years. But we can't. People are more stressed out than ever before. Rates of burnout are on the rise and many experts are warning of a mental-health tsunami around the corner.

We too often forget that mind and body are not just 'connected' – *our mind is a part of our body*. This is why living an unhappy life can have serious consequences for both our mental wellbeing *and* our physical health. Little by little, often without us even realizing, stresses build up inside us. Every time we get frustrated with another human being or wish things were different from the way they are, we bring tension into our body. Every time we get annoyed at a colleague's email, leave a negative comment on someone else's social media profile or look down on another human being, we bring tension into the body. Over time this tension builds up and we experience a lack of ease in our bodies. And what do we call a lack of ease in the body? Dis-ease. Lack of ease becomes disease.

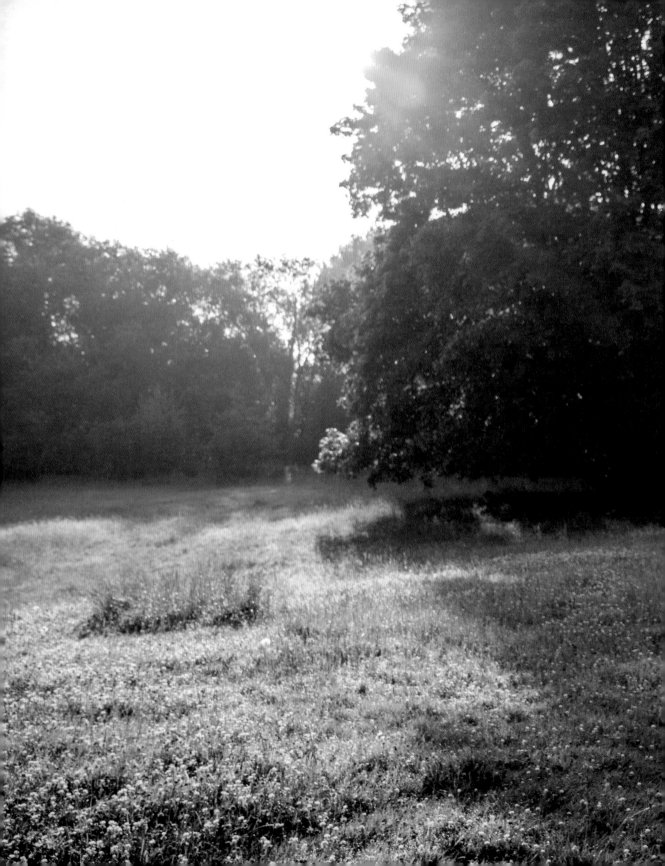

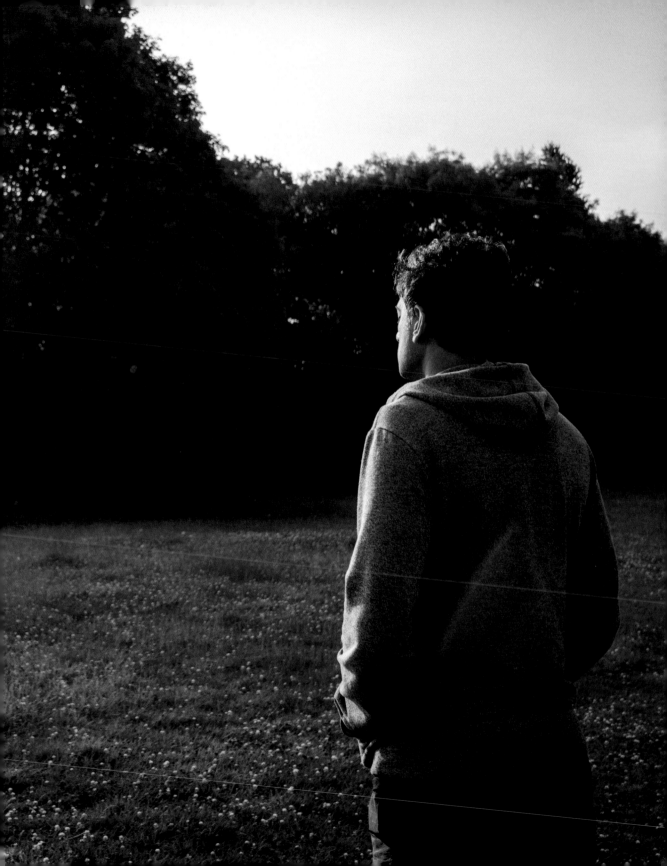

CORE HAPPINESS

People have been debating the nature of happiness since at least the days of Ancient Greece, 2,500 years ago. These arguments still continue, and will probably never be over, but based on my years of research in this area, and my hands-on experience of dealing with patients in the real world, I've come up with a new definition of happiness that I've seen to be accurate and genuinely useful, time and time again. I've designed this unique model of happiness specifically so that it can be practised and strengthened over time. I call it Core Happiness.

Core Happiness is not about bouncing out of bed every morning, all grins, sparkles and fairy dust. It's not about the peak experiences of joy you might feel on Christmas morning with the kids or when you step off a flight abroad and feel that glorious first blast of sun on your face. It's about moving your baseline level of happiness upwards so that you feel negative emotions less often, and for shorter bursts. It's about developing a resilient bubble of happiness around you that offers protection from the inevitable stresses and strains of life. It's about making sure your happiness isn't overly dependent on other people or external events. It's about treating happiness as you'd treat your physical body, making it stronger with smart and effective regular practice.

So how does it work? You can picture Core Happiness as a three-legged stool. Each of the legs is separate, but essential. If one of them is knocked away, your feelings of happiness will probably collapse. The first leg of the stool is contentment. Feeling content means being at peace with your life and your decisions. The second leg is control. Being in control means that you feel able to make meaningful decisions and that nothing, within reason, has the power to overwhelm you. The third leg is alignment. Feeling aligned means that the person you want to be, and the person you are actually being out there in the world, are one and the same. You're aligned when your inner values and your day-to-day actions match up.

CORE HAPPINESS AS A THREE-LEGGED STOOL

You can picture Core Happiness as a three-legged stool. Each of the legs is separate, but essential. If one of them is knocked away, your feelings of happiness will probably collapse.

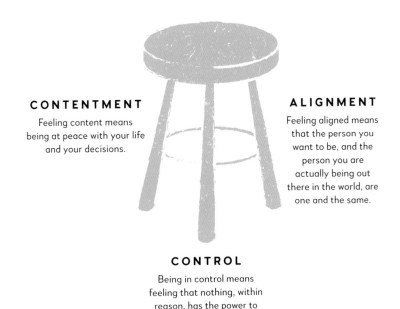

CONTENTMENT

Feeling content means being at peace with your life and your decisions.

ALIGNMENT

Feeling aligned means that the person you want to be, and the person you are actually being out there in the world, are one and the same.

CONTROL

Being in control means feeling that nothing, within reason, has the power to overwhelm you.

The important thing to remember about Core Happiness is that it isn't a final destination you'll one day reach, and then everything will be pure joy for ever. This is a journey. The three-legged stool doesn't stay upright all the time for anyone. Some days will be better than other days. But with regular practice, your Core Happiness stool will certainly become more stable. If you want bigger muscles, you've got to do resistance training regularly. Core Happiness works the same way. You must feed the part of you that you want to grow. And I promise you, it's absolutely worth it. The stronger your Core Happiness is, the closer you'll move to being that happy, carefree person you once were.

JUNK HAPPINESS

When our Core Happiness takes a hit, and that stool topples over, it hurts. Feeling out of control, discontented or out of alignment creates negative emotions that we'll instinctively try to run away from in any way we can. Usually we'll reach for the nearest and quickest solution – something that makes us feel a bit less unhappy, even if it's a short-term fix. I call this Junk Happiness. We all have a go-to Junk Happiness habit, something that we use to numb the inevitable pain of living. It could be a glass of wine, chocolate, Instagram or online shopping. When I was a young man, one of my Junk Happiness habits was gambling. The thrill of risking more money than I could afford on football, golf, a game of pool – in fact, anything – would enable me to forget my worries in the here and now, but always at a cost to my Core Happiness in the long term.

I'm not saying that these pleasures are always bad. The problem comes when we engage in these behaviours regularly and find ourselves reaching for Junk Happiness too often. Another comes when we use these treats not as occasional pleasures but to try to fill the hole inside us that's created by a lack of Core Happiness. The difference between Core and Junk Happiness is in the intention. Drinking a glass of wine when you're out in a bar connecting with friends isn't the same as drinking half a bottle by yourself because you're lonely. It's the same drug, but the intention is different.

One of the ways you can tell Core from Junk Happiness is how you feel when you remember it. When you recall engaging in a behaviour, does it fill you up with happiness all over again? Or does it make you shrink? If that alcohol you enjoyed with your friends makes you feel bigger when you remember it, it was probably nourishing you and building Core Happiness. But if the memory makes you shrink inside, it was almost certainly Junk.

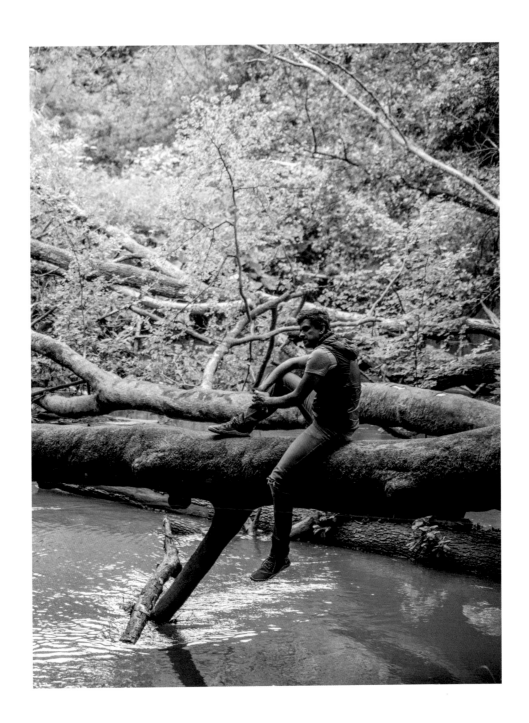

ALL THE HAPPINESS YOU NEED IS ALREADY INSIDE YOU

The aim of this book is to help you become the architect of your own happiness and health. I want to move you back towards that happier version of you we imagined at the beginning. You still possess all the raw ingredients for happiness. At its root, happiness is a feeling and, like any feeling, it's the result of the action of various chemicals that move through your brain and body. Technically, it's the result of chemicals like dopamine, oxytocin, endorphins, endocannabinoids and gamma aminobutyric acid. As long as you're physically capable of producing these incredible chemicals, the potential for happiness is there.

What stops you producing these chemicals and feeling all the happiness you desire? The stresses and strains of everyday life are clearly a large part of the answer. But, despite what you might assume, you don't need all of these stresses to magically disappear in order to feel happy. In fact, not only is this unnecessary, it's impossible.

So, if getting rid of all our stresses and pressures is not the secret of happiness, what is? Some of the smartest words I've ever read on happiness are by the psychologist Professor Daniel Nettle: 'Happiness stems mainly not from the world itself, but from the way people address the world.' This is one of the few things in life you can work on directly. You have all the resources you need to do it available to you already. It's about making internal, not external, changes, so in the pages that follow I'm going to introduce you to a new and practical way of approaching your life.

I want to show you that happiness is something anyone can grow with the right kind of practice. This fact alone should be cause for a smile. Just as if you eat a lot of chocolate you'll put on weight, and if you do daily bicep curls you'll develop bigger arms, if you follow the advice in this book, you will inevitably become happier. And, as you become happier, you *will* become healthier as well. You'll sleep better, feel calmer and experience more joy. You'll also find it much easier to take care of yourself and eat well.

Some people argue that any focus on a personal responsibility for happiness is wrong, because it takes attention away from all the wider problems we have in society, such as poverty, discrimination and social mobility. I completely agree that there is a lot in society that makes life harder for some people, especially for marginalized groups and those who struggle financially. I want society to change. But I can't wait for that to happen. You can't wait for that to happen. I've felt a powerful calling to write a book that can help you no matter who you are.

CHOOSE HAPPY

Every one of these chapters is based on a combination of cutting-edge science, and my decades of experience as a doctor and a human being. They contain universal principles that cost little or nothing to practise, that you can apply in your own life right now. They don't require you to put yourself through a dramatic life reboot. You don't even have to follow them all.

Everyone's route to happiness is different and your happiness prescription is going to be different from mine. But, by the end of the book, you will definitely feel empowered to write your very own happiness prescription – one that is perfect for you and *your* life.

The magical thing about happiness is that it's a subjective feeling: if you feel happy, you are happy. And every day you have the ability to make simple decisions that enable you to feel happier, more of the time. In other words: happiness is a decision.

I can't change the fact that you'll encounter problems and stresses in your day-to-day life. But I can change how you feel about them. All you need to do is decide.

So, what's your decision? Do you want to be happy? Do you want to be healthier? Do you want to flow through life with ease and calm? If so, read on.

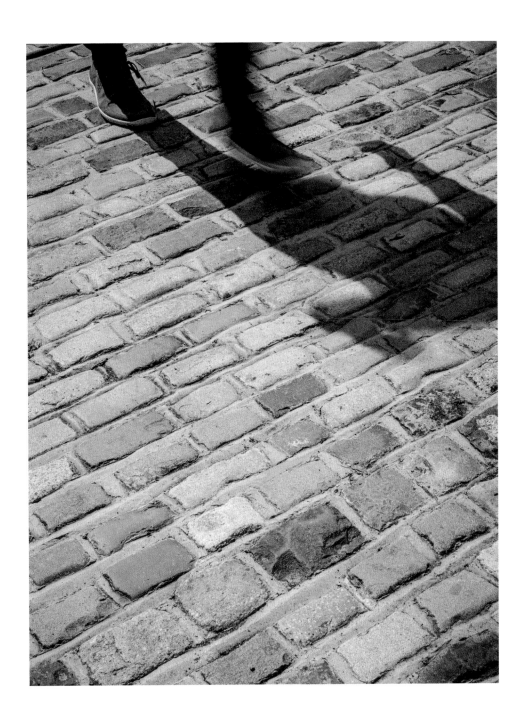

№ 1

WRITE YOUR
HAPPY ENDING

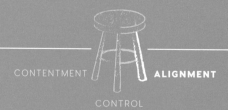

CONTENTMENT   ALIGNMENT

CONTROL

One of the biggest obstacles to people increasing their happiness is that they often misunderstand what it actually is. They think they need a nicer car, a more exotic holiday or a fancier job title to become happier. But you don't need to buy *anything* to access happiness, or to go to some other country. Happiness isn't about money or material goods. Neither is it about class, colour, sexuality, social media followers or career achievement. I know many wealthy doctors, lawyers and CEOs who are utterly miserable. And I know many people on much more modest incomes who are intensely happy and satisfied with their lives.

The problem, in a nutshell, is that we mistake success for happiness. I believe that for most people the single biggest reason they're walking around with a hole in their heart which they try unsuccessfully to fill with a whole host of compensatory behaviours – such as alcohol, junk food, sugar and overwork – is because they've made this fundamental error. From a tender age, we are taught that in order to thrive we need to be better than the people around us. We can only be successful if it comes at the expense of others. We are given the impression that in order to succeed at life we need to excel in our exams, so we can get a better job and earn more money. This is how happiness is defined for us. Society takes us as soon as it can and puts us through its brainwashing programme. Don't get me wrong, I've got nothing against success. But success is *not* the same thing as happiness.

YOUR DREAMS WON'T
MAKE YOU HAPPY

In 1962, my dad travelled from India to Britain, hoping for a better life. My mother joined him in 1972. Dad was one of eight children and, after training as a doctor at Calcutta National Medical College, he decided to leave for the UK to give his family more opportunities. He became a brilliant surgeon in obstetrics and gynaecology, and ended up as a consultant at Manchester Royal Infirmary in a different specialty. A few years before he died, he said to me, 'You know, son, when I was a child I could never have dreamed of owning my own house or my own car. In India, you can work hard and never get such rewards. I knew if I worked hard in England, I would reap the benefits.' My dad worked hard. He earned enough to have nice holidays and send his kids to private school. But he was not happy.

In his dogged pursuit of success, my dad slept just three nights a week. I remember him coming home from work every evening at about five thirty. He'd shower and shave, Mum would give him dinner and then a car would pick him up at six forty-five. He'd then spend all night doing GP calls and seeing patients. He'd come in again at 7 a.m., shave, drive into Manchester and work all day. That was his life for thirty years. It's one of the main reasons why he got diagnosed with the auto-immune disease lupus at fifty-nine, went on to develop kidney failure and ended up on dialysis for fifteen years, which forced him into early retirement.

Despite his brilliance and his exceptionally hard work, my dad was unfairly held back by racist attitudes that were, sadly, extremely widespread at the time. He'd train all the 'local' doctors in surgery and, within two or three years, they'd have jumped over him on the career ladder and usually be promoted as he was left behind. This happened for years. In order to give his family security and make consultant grade, he reluctantly gave up his dream job as a surgeon and moved to

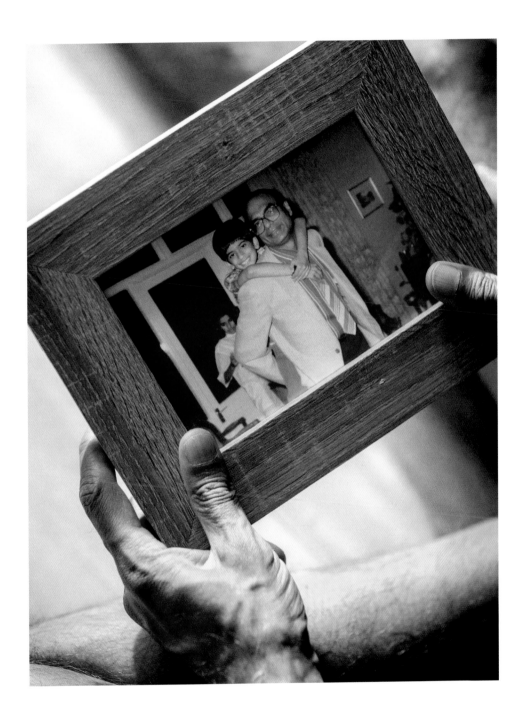

a less popular specialty that he didn't really enjoy. He never complained to me about this when I was young, confiding how heartbreaking he found it only when he was on his deathbed.

The stresses that came with his relentless and challenging pursuit of success created tensions at home. My mum dealt with it by numbing herself with TV soap operas every night – *Coronation Street, Brookside, EastEnders, The Bold and the Beautiful, Hart to Hart*, the lot. It's probably fair to say she was addicted to them. When she went on holiday she'd make sure they were all taped for her to binge when she got back. These days, of course, she'd probably be glued to Instagram, TikTok or Facebook.

Like a lot of immigrants, my parents traded in the raw ingredients of happiness for those of success. Back in India, they'd have enjoyed the benefits of a loving, supportive community, extended family and as much help with the kids as they needed. There would have been no prejudice against them. Despite the success they made of life in Britain, they were still unhappy. I believe a lot of immigrants come to regret the trade they make. They fall for this widespread but utterly false idea of what happiness is – the house, the car, the holiday. My parents brought me up to believe in it too. I grew up thinking that success and coming top of the class and getting a great job mattered above anything else. As a child, I hated losing. If I lost at Ludo, I'd have a tantrum and storm out of the room. And when I won? Of course I'd feel happy for a short time. But the win just made the desire to win again next time even greater – and the pain of loss fiercer.

We're told to follow our dreams. We devote our lives to chasing them, and make sacrifice after sacrifice in order to make them all come true. But what we're never told is this: our dreams won't make us happy.

MEET THE WANT BRAIN

Perhaps the most surprising thing about this myth of happiness is just how many people wholeheartedly believe in it. I'd bet that the majority of people around the world would be surprised to hear that achieving their dreams won't make them happy – and many would be offended, perhaps criticizing me for making such a cynical-sounding statement. The reason the myth is so easy to fall for is that it directly connects with a part of the brain that scientists call the 'system of desire'. This system of desire, which operates on mid-brain dopamine circuits, is extremely powerful. It was designed by evolution at a time when food and other resources were often scarce. It motivates us to compete with other people and grab as much for ourselves and for our family as we can. It's not interested in our happiness. Instead, it's programmed to make us think and behave in such a way that we maximize our chances of survival. It's incredibly strong because it's a relic of a time when those chances often weren't very good and life expectancy for an adult was around thirty.

I call this system the Want Brain. It's that part of you that is utterly convinced that a slab of chocolate, a bigger television or a promotion at work will make you happy, and it tells you this is true multiple times a day. One of the reasons we know this is a lie is because of clever research that involves contacting people at random times of the day, asking what they're doing, then asking how they feel. The consistent but surprising result is that activities the Want Brain sells us as 'fun', such as eating chocolate, watching television or moseying around the shops, actually leave us feeling less motivated, less confident and more depressed.

When you're under the spell of the Want Brain, tens of thousands of years of evolution are whispering in your ear and plotting against you. It is quite literally Stone Age thinking, and it's probably responsible for more daily unhappiness, in the modern age, than wars or pandemics. I've seen the damage it can do myself.

LIVING IN A WANT BRAIN WORLD

Our whole society is set up around the satisfaction of all our wants. We want a great job, we want a great car, we want a great holiday, we want a great house. And in order to get all that we desire, we want money. The Western world is a market economy. This means that, in order to keep itself functional, it has to have as many of its citizens as possible making and circulating as much money as possible. To achieve this, the Want Brain must be constantly stimulated and encouraged. We're tempted by advertising and the continual cycle of new products that come into the shops – the latest phone, the latest fashions, the hottest destinations. We're encouraged to equate professional success with happiness. Society itself conspires with our Want Brains to make us truly believe these trinkets will make us happy. No wonder all our hearts are broken.

My full indoctrination into Want Brain culture probably began when I was seven. My parents took me to Midland Bank with a cheque for £10, which I used to open a Griffin Saver bank account. I was given a dictionary, my own paying-in book that looked like a chequebook and a smart blue folder. I even had a Griffin Saver badge that I proudly pinned on to my school blazer. I felt like such a grown-up. What was all this telling me? That being a grown-up was about money. And to make money, I had to be a success. This indoctrination continued at school, where I was repeatedly given the impression that life was all about passing exams with flying colours so I could get the job of my dreams. All of this spoke directly to my Want Brain. As a result, I made winning my identity. Ninety-nine per cent was never good enough for me – and it wasn't good enough for my parents either. Only 100 per cent would do.

We don't realize we're doing it, but we all sign an adulthood contract. This contract says that we're going to contribute to the market economy by making and spending as much money as possible. So, we leave school and get a job and expect this kind of success to make us happy. But it doesn't. So we strive to get the next promotion, thinking this will finally make us happy. We realize that we're still unhappy. We don't understand it. We're doing everything that's asked of us but life feels empty. We ask ourselves, why? And we're so indoctrinated into the Want Brain mindset that we think: if I'm unhappy, it must be because I'm still not making enough money. So back on the treadmill we go. I know so many 'successful' professionals like this. They're not short of cash, they have a nice house and a nice car, but they're miserable. They hate their job. They went into it because their parents wanted them to. By the time they hit their mid-thirties they're married with a mortgage and often have school fees to pay. They're feeding the economy and are outwardly a 'success'. But the truth is, they're trapped. And, to compensate for the pain, they drink to excess every weekend.

Of course, these kinds of feelings aren't exclusive to high earners like bankers and lawyers. I can't count the number of patients I've seen who get seduced by Want Brain thinking. They're trapped in a futile attempt to become happier by working themselves into the ground, chasing a bigger car, a better holiday or a flashier phone and are unsuccessfully trying to make themselves feel better by impressing others. Trying to increase your self-worth by gaining the acceptance of others is always destined in failure. It never lasts, it doesn't deal with the root of the problem and relying on it has a negative impact on our mental and physical health.

I am not saying that money has no relationship at all to happiness. Much of the research in this area suggests that once we have enough money to cover our basic needs, like food and shelter, more money does not actually make us significantly happier. And, if we think about the Core Happiness stool, we can see that money, depending on our current situation, has the potential to help us gain a sense of control and autonomy over our lives. But, as a society, I think we vastly over-emphasize the importance of money. Money removes common sources of unhappiness. But it does not bring us happiness in and of itself. True happiness comes from within.

To see how unnatural and unhealthy the modern world has become, we can compare how we live today, with our Want Brains being constantly stimulated, to how we used to live. The things we do for pleasure, in the twenty-first century, we once did for survival. Our 'job' used to involve fishing, hunting, foraging or cooking. Men might go on a hunt, walking and chatting with their buddies on the way, engaging in the companionship and buzz of the shared mission. They'd be out in nature, moving their body. The women would also spend much of their time with friends and relatives, chatting and laughing and picking tubers, nuts and berries. At night the whole tribe would gather together round the campfire, gossiping, telling stories and singing. There are still indigenous tribes around the world, like the Hadza tribe in Tanzania, who live like this – in harmony with nature and themselves.

Of course, I'm not saying every aspect of life was perfect in our past – far from it. Much has improved in our modern lives. But not everything has. Today, modern humans pay good money to do the things we once did as our daily work. We still enjoy these pastimes today because we're designed to enjoy them. They're the things that humans are supposed to do. We're not wired to sit in an office all day, or behind the wheel of a taxi, or spend hours in a stuffy commuter train. When we're unhappy in these situations, we often think there's something wrong with us. But there isn't. If you put a member of the northern Tanzanian Hadza tribe in an office for eight hours, they'd be miserable too. Your unhappiness is an entirely rational response to the madness of the modern world.

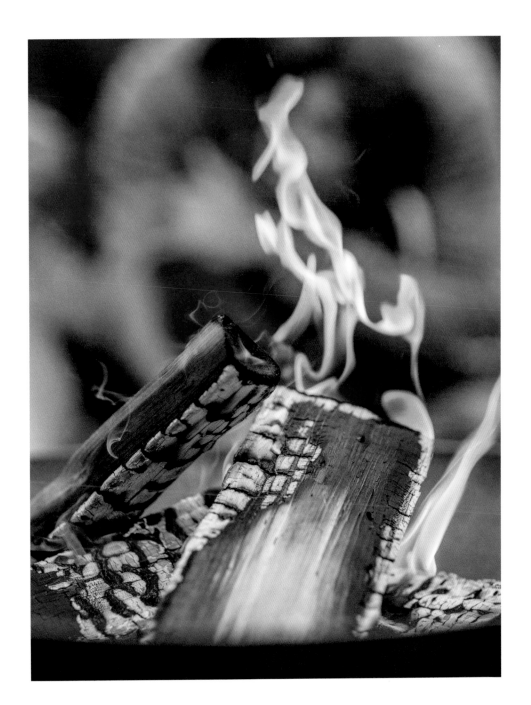

Redefine success

When we define success, we also define failure. If we decide that a properly lived life is one in which all our material desires are met – like having the perfect sofa for our living room, planning the 'perfect' birthday party for our kids, eating at the latest restaurant and subsequently posting about it on social media, etc. – we've also decided that when we don't manage to constantly 'win', we're a failure. This is a recipe for misery. Once we've signed the adulthood contract, we've scripted our own unhappiness. The answer? Redefine success.

When the Want Brain has control of us, we can so easily forget the simple pleasures in life that can truly make us happy, such as having a relaxing bath or a walk in nature. One of my favourite things to do on a Sunday afternoon, after I've cleaned up the kitchen, is to put on a Ray LaMontagne CD (yes, I still listen to CDs and you'll shortly find out why!) and make butternut squash soup for two hours. I'm literally in heaven. It doesn't matter if I've had a brilliant week at work or it's been incredibly stressful, for those two hours, I'm king of the world.

In the iconic *Tao Te Ching* it says, 'knowing what is enough is wealth'. This is exactly what this entire 'redefining success' process is about: deciding what is enough and using that to define what a successful week and life really looks like. This is not about earning more money, getting a promotion at work or buying a new toy. This is about things that truly bring you happiness and bypass the Want Brain.

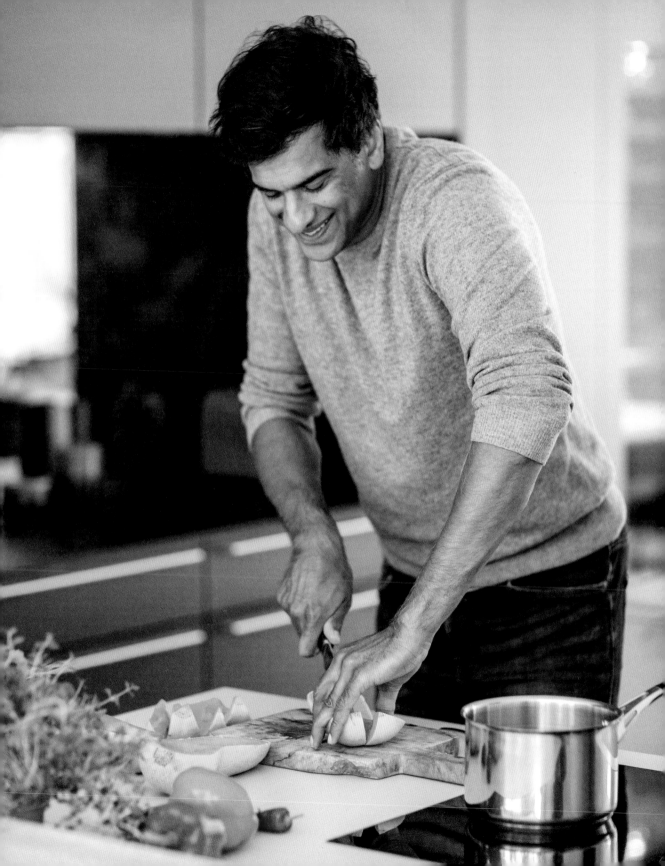

DEFINE YOUR HAPPINESS HABITS

- Write down three things that give you an intense feeling of wellbeing: let's call them Happiness Habits. See if you can do them all each week. For example, a successful week for you might include a walk in nature, an Epsom Salt bath and three meals at the table with your family. Or it might be spending time with one of your close friends, time to play your guitar and going out for lunch with your mum. Your Happiness Habits will be unique to you.

- Over time, you can increase the number of Happiness Habits slowly but surely. You may not manage to do them all every week but the practice of defining them and assessing how many you've done will help you counteract the happiness-killing effects of the Want Brain world.

WRITE YOUR HAPPY ENDING

- Now take a moment to write down what a happy life looks like for you. Imagine you're on your deathbed. Looking back, what are the three most important things you will want to have done in order to feel happy and content? This is an incredibly useful exercise as it helps give you a 30,000-foot view on the direction of your life.

- Understanding these big, overarching life goals will help you to shape your daily and weekly Happiness Habits. For me, I'll be happy at the end of my life if I've contributed to the wellbeing of others; spent undistracted time with my friends and family; and had time to focus on activities that I'm passionate about. So, on a weekly basis, if I manage to record an episode of my podcast, have regular sit-down meals with my family and find time to play my guitar or a bit of snooker, I know that I'm living more intentionally and moving in the right direction.

Doing these two simple exercises regularly will help you to redefine success for yourself. The 'Define Your Happiness Habits' exercise is a great one to do on a weekly basis, perhaps on a Sunday morning over a cup of tea. The 'Write Your Happy Ending' one can be done more infrequently – perhaps monthly or quarterly.

These exercises are about bringing a heightened awareness to your life and how you're living it. It's only through this awareness that you bring about the possibility of change.

Once you define what success looks like for you, you'll find that you start to move your focus on to the right things, turning down the noise from your Want Brain and increasing the volume on happiness.

REDEFINE YOURSELF

How you identify is incredibly important to happiness. I'm so much happier than I was five years ago because I've been through a conscious process of getting rid of my labels. Most labels are fictional and are given to us by society. According to society, I'm a doctor and I'm a father. On the surface, this may not seem problematic, but I've learned that these ideas are more troublesome than they seem. Without being consciously aware of it, they often result in us trying to live in accordance with how we think these identities *should* live.

If we become too strongly attached to our labels, they can leave us feeling fragile and exposed. If we were to lose them, for any reason, we'd lose our sense of who we are. Take my label as a 'doctor'. What if I got sick and was unable to work any longer? What if I got fired from my job? Who would I be then? How would I feel about myself if my whole identity was wrapped up in the idea of being a doctor and I could no longer be one? This often happens when people retire. Their happiness and their health start to go downhill because they've lost their sense of self.

And what about my label as a father? It seems like something to be intensely proud of. And, to be really clear, my job as a father is one of the most important roles in my life. I'm determined to be the best father I can, and I aspire to bring up my children to be kind, compassionate human beings. But being a good father is not who I am. It's simply a role that I play. If I get too attached to that label, what happens if my kids were to get annoyed and tell me I'm a bad parent? What happens when they get older and leave home? If I am too strongly attached to the identity of being a father, I run the risk of spiralling into the trap of Junk Happiness. These days, I no longer define myself as a doctor or as a father, but as a curious human. This identity holds true for me in every role I play in life and works no matter what situation I find myself in. Understanding this has given me a deep sense of freedom and peace.

Identity Menu

I'd like you to begin the process of redefining who you are. Your personal identity comes from your values. So what do you truly value in life? Below I've listed some possible values to help you start. This is not an exhaustive list, so use it as a guide only and feel free to add your own.

- Curiosity
- Integrity
- Compassion
- Family
- Creativity
- Honesty
- The climate and the planet

- Solitude
- Nature
- Wisdom
- Conscientiousness
- Standing up for other people
- Humility
- Kindness

- Loyalty
- Self-respect
- Intimacy
- Time for friends and family
- Empathy
- Being a good listener

To start with, I'd like you to choose three values. Every week, take a moment to assess how you're doing in becoming that person. I'd recommend that you write your values down somewhere to help you set your intention and to help keep you accountable. Perhaps, like me, you could put your values at the top of your social media profile. Or you could pop them on a Post-it note and stick it on your fridge. The act of doing this exercise, writing them down and putting them somewhere visible is incredibly beneficial.

This is your first step to happiness. It's crucial because you're not going to get 'there' if you haven't first defined where 'there' is. When you assess how you're doing every week, don't be too harsh on yourself. This is going to be a lifelong journey. All we are looking for is increased awareness and steady improvement.

WHY ALIGNMENT MATTERS

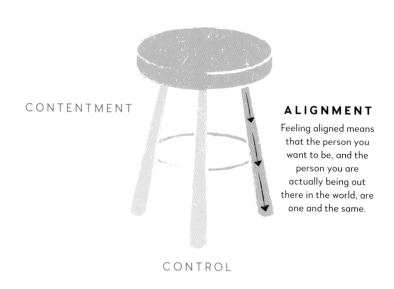

CONTENTMENT

ALIGNMENT
Feeling aligned means
that the person you
want to be, and the
person you are
actually being out
there in the world, are
one and the same.

CONTROL

This process of consciously defining your identity is critically important because it helps strengthen the alignment leg of the Core Happiness stool. Alignment is when your inner values and external actions match up. But how do you know how aligned you are if you've never taken time to define what your values are in the first place? The 'Identity Menu' exercise is incredibly powerful and designed to trigger this process, by allowing you to consciously assess your internal values. Once you have done this, you are then able to assess if your day-to-day behaviours match up with them.

Do you say that you value undistracted time with your family, yet your real-world evidence shows that you hardly have any at all? Do you say that you value your health, yet, on reflection, can never find time for self-care? Do you say that you value being kind but, after honest assessment, realize that you have been a little

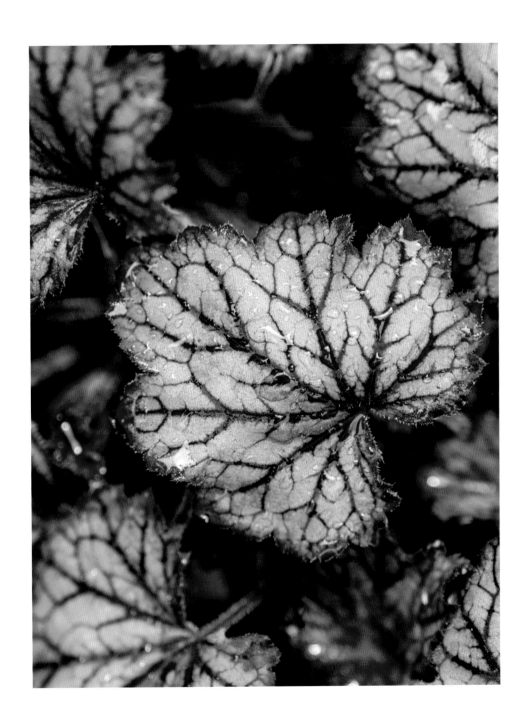

ELIMINATE CHOICE

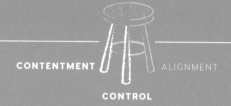

CONTENTMENT ALIGNMENT

CONTROL

Every Saturday night, once the kids were safely in bed, my wife, Vidh, and I used to settle down on the couch downstairs to watch a film. We'd usually flick to Netflix, because they had the most choice. With the remote in hand, we'd move through all the options – New Releases, Classics, Drama, True Crime, Biopics. How about a documentary? Hmm, what were we in the mood for? We'd weigh up all the choices, and start to disagree. We try to find a compromise. After about forty-five minutes, with our moods spoilt, we'd usually decide to just forget about it and end up watching nothing.

One of the apparently marvellous things about the modern age is the number of choices it offers us. The Want Brain world we live in is designed to offer as many options as possible, wherever possible: in shops, restaurants, in the media and online. When we come to book our holiday, pretty much the entire planet is open to us, as long as we have the funds. We can even go on a trip to North Korea, if we fancy it. Studies suggest we make an astonishing 35,000 choices every day, with 226.7 decisions made on food alone. We rarely stop to ask ourselves, is this overwhelming choice actually good for us? If you could transport Vidh and me back in time to an England that had only three television channels, would we enjoy happier Saturday nights at home and achieve more connection? The answer, almost certainly, is yes.

THE CHOICE TRAP

Too much choice brings major happiness downsides. Every day, every single decision we make takes something from us. Each one takes cognitive effort. Each one takes time. And our peace of mind, because the more options we're given, the less confident we'll be that we've made the very best one. Researchers know that shops who offer too much choice cause their customers to feel stressed. If supermarkets offer twenty-eight flavours of a product, its sales plummet. But if they offer only three, sales go through the roof. Deciding between three options usually isn't overwhelming, but being faced with twenty-eight means people are almost certainly going to be left with a nagging feeling of anxiety. Similarly, psychologists find that if we're given the option of taking an item of clothing back to the shop to swap, it makes us less happy and confident in our purchase, once again damaging our state of mind.

We associate choice with freedom. In fact, we often treat choice and freedom as if they're the same thing. In most societies, we treat freedom as if it's a sacred right, but the freedom to choose a Prime Minister to lead a nation isn't the same as being made to choose between seventy-two different yoghurts every time you go to the supermarket. To understand why, and to understand why being overwhelmed with choice, day after day, is guaranteed to make us miserable, we need to revisit our new friend, the Core Happiness stool.

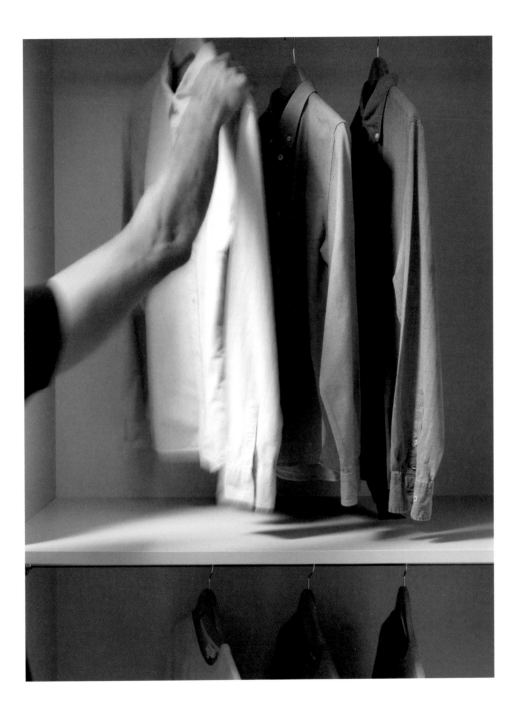

FALSE VERSUS MEANINGFUL CHOICES

The anxiety and doubt created by being faced with too many decisions kicks away two legs of the Core Happiness stool, making us feel less content and less in control of the world. Part of the practice of building Core Happiness is calming down the Want Brain. But when we're continually presented with choice after choice, it gets fed and becomes stronger. The Want Brain is always taking us to a place of 'what if?' It makes us doubt our choices and feeds our insecurities. The Want Brain makes us continually wonder, 'Could my life be a bit better if I made a different choice?' The more unsure we become, the less content and in control we feel, the more our Core Happiness is weakened.

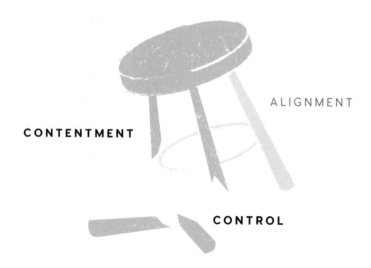

CONTENTMENT

ALIGNMENT

CONTROL

But living a life without any choice at all wouldn't just be impossible, it would be unbelievably dull. To hit the right balance, it's helpful to get good at spotting the difference between false and meaningful choices.

One of the ultimate meaningful choices that some of us choose to make is that of our marriage partner. When we choose a lover for life, and say our vows, we're telling the world that we've made our decision for ever. One of the hidden joys of marriage is that it radically eliminates future choices, meaning we can simply stop thinking about others in a romantic way. This strengthens your Core Happiness by helping you feel more content and gives you heightened sense of control, as life feels more predictable.

Marriage is clearly a different kind of decision to, say, choosing a bottle of wine in a restaurant. If you're a wine buff and you build Core Happiness by thinking about wine, that's great. You'll make an informed choice and probably be satisfied with it. But, if you're not, agonizing over which wine to order is not going to make you happy. Instead, you're more likely to experience it as a moment of anxiety. You might beat yourself up a little for not knowing what to pick, then regret the choice you do finally end up with. You'll experience the decision in a completely different way to the connoisseur, to whom pondering the wine list may be a high point of the evening.

If the non-connoisseur feels anxious about their wine order, they've allowed themselves to become tripped up by a false choice. It's false because, no matter which bottle they order, they'll surely enjoy it. In fact, they probably won't be able to tell much difference between the various bottles on offer. When psychologists test wine experts under laboratory conditions, they find they struggle to tell the difference even between red and white wine. Many of the choices we make in day-to-day life are just like this – false choices that actually take more happiness from us than they offer. We can build Core Happiness by choosing only when it matters and when, once we've chosen, we accept our decisions.

TOO MUCH CHOICE
AFFECTS OUR HEALTH

A few years back, I attended a lifestyle medicine conference in America. At lunchtime, I nipped out to a local food stall. I just wanted a salmon salad but was asked about ten questions along the way – What size? Would I like berries on it? Would I like sauce? If so, what sauce? Would I like pickles, tomatoes, what kind of tomatoes, and so on. Yes, I got my healthy salad, but I also got a major side order of stress, which will have undone many of the benefits of the food.

If there's one thing that life in a twenty-first-century Want Brain world guarantees, it's stress. Every day, from the very moment we awake, we're assailed by what I call Micro Stress Doses. This is a concept I introduced in my second book, *The Stress Solution*, which really struck a chord with my readers. I think it is worth touching on again as it beautifully illustrates how too much choice can impact our health.

Micro Stress Doses (MSDs) are the tiny moments of anxiety, frustration or fear we get from watching the news or seeing something triggering on social media, or from leaving the house late and having to deal with heavy traffic and a toddler kicking the back of our seat for the journey's duration. In isolation, we can usually cope with MSDs just fine. The problem comes when they start to build up. The more MSDs we absorb in a day, the closer we'll be pushed to our own personal stress threshold. This is the point at which we feel like we can't take any more. When we cross our stress threshold we become reactive, emotional and angry. Our necks might go into spasm, our backs start to seize up, our migraines get triggered or our IBS symptoms flare.

Working too much, long commutes, inadequate sleep and emotional tensions can all of course contribute to daily stress loads. But so can too much choice. Every time you make an unnecessary choice, you're creating tension and stress in your mind and body. Every time you can't decide what film to watch, which song to listen to, which meal to order at the restaurant, which book to choose at the bookshop, which podcast to listen to, which model of phone to buy, you are adding to your day's stress load. And, little by little, this is taking you closer and closer to your personal stress threshold. It's impossible to be happy when we're near our threshold. We feel out of control, discontent and, when the next MSD arrives, we're almost certainly going to act out of alignment. The problem was not the last MSD, it was the build-up throughout the day.

In isolation, each of these choices may not feel like much, but I can assure you, from my clinical and personal experience, these stress doses add up very quickly. I firmly believe that too much choice is one of the main reasons most of us are walking around feeling burned out, overwhelmed, tired and stressed out, with knock-on consequences for our wellbeing. Chronic, unrelenting stress can cause or contribute to many different health problems, including insomnia, anxiety, depression, gut problems, hormone problems, autoimmune problems, heart disease and brain degeneration.

I want to liberate you from the weight of your MSDs and the problems they cause. Reducing unnecessary choice is an amazingly effective way to do this.

 (To hear a podcast conversation where I talk in depth about Micro Stress Doses and the impact of stress on our health, visit drchatterjee.com/41.)

CASE STUDY

It's not uncommon for me to see the damage that too much choice has on my patients. Forty-year-old Martin came to see me after experiencing breathlessness and chest pain when going up stairs. After tests and investigations, I realized the pain was coming from his heart. He was shocked and determined to do something about it but was adamant that he did not want any medication.

Martin led a pretty sedentary lifestyle and agreed to start regular exercise. But when I saw him a few months later, he still hadn't started doing anything. He told me he couldn't decide what to do. One of his mates was into triathlons, another did weights down the gym and another still swore running had been life-changing for him. Martin had spent months researching the 'best' form of exercise to do. Ironically, all this research was done while he sat down in front of his laptop. Simply having to make the choice had been paralysing for him and, on some nights, this even affected his sleep as he felt so confused.

I asked him what he thought he could get cracking on with without doing much research. He said walking. 'Great,' I replied. 'Can you commit to a fifteen-minute walk every day at the same time?' He agreed to do this at eight o'clock every morning. As his health improved, and his chest pains eased, he gained motivation and built up momentum. After a few months, he had built up to forty-five minutes each day. This had a knock-on effect to other areas of his life. He ended up eating better and prioritizing his sleep more. He realized how too much choice was affecting him in other areas of his life and started to write weekly meal plans to reduce meal stress. He loved listening to health podcasts and, on my advice, decided to stick to just one or two instead of being overwhelmed every time he opened up his podcast app.

A year later, he was unrecognizable. His heart health had improved to the point where he no longer experienced any chest pains, but he was also much happier. He felt more in control of his life, more content and more aligned. Of course, the walking will have helped his overall health, but the reduction in stress he experienced by eliminating choice would've also had a significant effect. If I hadn't pushed him to eliminate choice, he'd never have seen these benefits to his health – or his happiness.

WAYS TO ELIMINATE CHOICE

Courtney Carver, a fashion executive, used to get overwhelmed by having to decide what to wear each morning. She decided to simplify the process by limiting her wardrobe choices. She called it Project 3–33. Courtney would dress with thirty-three items for three months, including clothes, accessories, jewellery and shoes, not counting underwear, sleepwear, at-home loungewear or work-out clothes.

The experience was life-changing. She learned that her closet was actually a major source of damage to her Core Happiness. She didn't have to be constantly knocked out of contentment by being reminded of poor purchases, clothes that didn't fit or that she did not like, or a wasteful purchase that still had its tags hanging off it. Project 3–33 became a movement, and now many more people are experiencing reduced stress and anxiety, more peaceful mornings, and are saving money and energy. Of course, there is also the additional benefit of helping the planet by not over-consuming limited resources and buying unnecessary clothes.

I've no doubt these people are benefiting from having their Core Happiness strengthened by feeling more in control and more content every morning. The secret at the core of Project 3–33 is eliminating choice. Once you've started to identify where you're regularly making false choices, you can start eliminating them. Music is one of my greatest loves. People often laugh at me because I still listen to CDs. I know many of us now just ask Alexa, but what I love about CDs is that the artist has decided for me what to listen to, and in which order. They've agonized over the very best track sequence possible. On a streaming service, you have access to every song that's been recorded in human history. You're drowning in false choices. If you find that you can never decide what to listen to, and regularly waste time and energy thinking about it, why not start listening to albums again?

Another way to eliminate choice is by making personal rules. For instance, if you're the kind of person who squints uncomfortably at the wine menu, why not make it a rule that you'll always buy the second-cheapest option? If you want to treat your family to a takeaway meal and no one can decide which restaurant to use, you could choose using dice or a game of Rock, Paper, Scissors. If you want to avoid agonizing over a new purchase, just ask someone you trust who knows what they're talking about and accept their advice. I used to be the kind of person who, when they wanted a new camera, would study the options for hours, comparing features and poring over each plus and minus. These days I just buy the first device someone recommends. All of the cameras on offer will do the job and do it well enough. I don't want to make the choice, so I don't.

You can add these rules in anywhere. Starbucks reportedly sells 80,000 different drinks combinations. It's the Alexa of the drinks world. Are you wasting energy, and eating away at Core Happiness, every time you go for a coffee? Would you benefit from always making one choice and sticking with it? Where else in your life are you choosing where you don't need to?

Save your energy for decisions that really matter.

Where can you eliminate choice in your life?

Where are you making unnecessary choices in your life? Where can you eliminate stress by reducing how many decisions you need to make?

Your lifestyle is unique to you and, therefore, the choices that really do matter to you will be different from those that matter to me. That is completely OK. What really matters is that we eliminate false choices wherever we can.

Use the following as examples to help you create your own personal choice rules.

- **Write a meal planner:** a major source of stress for many of us is deciding what we're going to cook and eat – planning your meals for the following week before doing your weekly shop helps remove this stress.

- **Choose a morning routine:** many of us become paralysed with choice and cannot decide which health habits to do each day, so end up doing nothing. Choose a morning routine that you think you will enjoy and do it. Don't constantly look for ways to change it or improve it. Doing something small regularly is better than doing nothing. See page 234 for more information on my own morning routine.

- **Create a film shortlist:** have a list of films in a journal or in an app on your phone. When it comes to film time, don't go through the streaming menu – just choose one from your personally curated list.

- **Be a selective listener:** only subscribe to one or two podcasts that give you the kind of topics you enjoy and the variety that you want. Then, instead of choosing between the millions of different podcasts on offer every time you open up the podcast app, you can start listening straight away.

- **Don't agonize over restaurant menus:** if you already know what you like, order it. Don't feel you have to add to your stress load every single time you eat out in a café or restaurant.

- **Pick a playlist:** listen to whole albums in the order the artist has created for you or allow a streaming service (such as Spotify, Apple or Amazon Music) to choose your playlist for you. These powerful computer algorithms are very good at learning your musical tastes from your previous listening habits. Let them take on the stress of choosing your playlist so you can just sit back and enjoy.

I would like you to do an audit of your own lifestyle and see where and how often you are making choices. Once you have done this, I want you to honestly ask yourself how many of these choices are really necessary. Create a personal list of rules where you will start to eliminate choice from your life. Don't worry about overhauling everything at once. Even one small change will start to yield results and you can build it up over time.

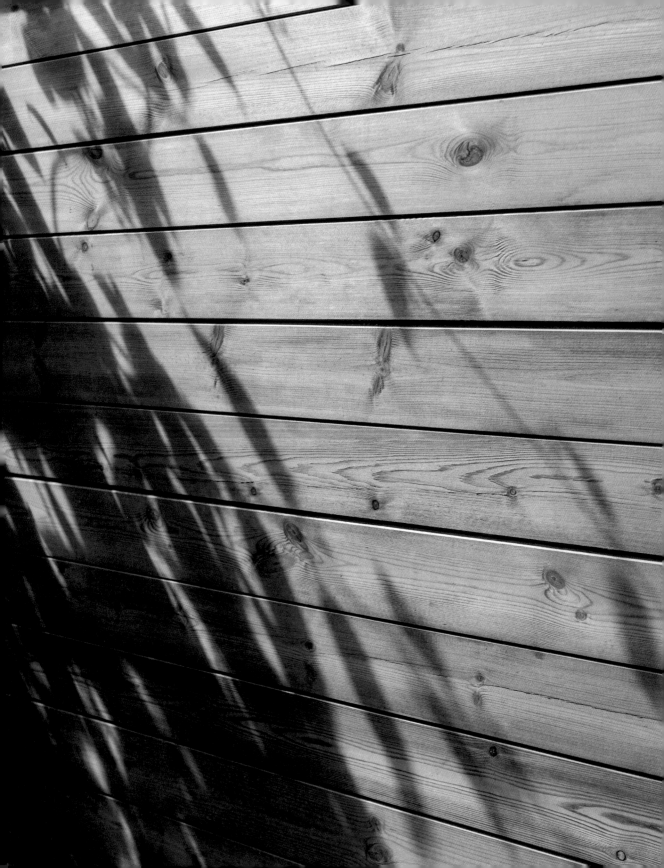

CONCLUSION

Too much choice is likely to be a massive hidden stressor in your life. It drains your cognitive energy and weakens your Core Happiness by making you feel less in control and less content. By eliminating choice, creating personal rules and adding routine, you're simplifying your life in ways that can transform both your health and your happiness.

№ 3

TREAT YOURSELF WITH RESPECT

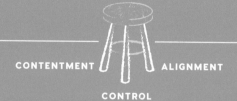

CONTENTMENT · ALIGNMENT

CONTROL

It's taken me many years to get my Want Brain under control. That little boy who would storm out of the lounge if he lost at Ludo grew into a young man who would physically attack himself whenever he felt like a failure. As a student at university in Edinburgh, I'd regularly play pool with my buddies. If the game wasn't going well, I'd go into the toilet, glare at myself in the mirror, call myself insulting names and then start slapping myself across the face. 'Come on, Chatterjee,' I'd shout. 'You're a loser.' I wanted so badly to win. More often than not, I did. But the cost of all that winning was self-loathing.

Many of us treat ourselves like this – with a chronic lack of respect. We live in a Want Brain world that tells us success and happiness are the same thing. We worry that if we're too kind to ourselves, we'll lose motivation, grow weak and fail at achieving our dreams. We make the same kinds of mistakes when we decide to change our lifestyles. Every January, during the season of New Year's resolutions, millions of us adopt a harsh deprivation–restriction mindset and begin punishing ourselves, mentally and physically. Yes, harsh tactics can often work for a few weeks. But the reason New Year's resolutions usually don't last is because they're coming not from a place of love, but a place of lack.

YOUR OWN WORST ENEMY

I've often reflected on the patients who managed to truly transform their lives for good. I'm talking about the people who came through my door with a set of physical symptoms and, by making changes to their lives, were able to not only improve their immediate issues but also their long-term health and happiness. The magic ingredient in these people wasn't their being especially motivated or rigorous in following my advice. It was that, somewhere along their journey, they'd simply started to like who they were. They practised self-compassion. Once they began treating themselves with respect, the changes they were trying to make no longer felt like a huge effort.

It's just not possible to achieve long-time health or happiness if you hate yourself. A person who truly loves who they are is unlikely to engage in self-sabotaging behaviours such as devouring a whole packet of chocolate biscuits or drinking alcohol to excess. The latest scientific research makes this clear. A 2020 study that surveyed the work of many researchers found a strong association between self-compassion and physical health. Self-compassion has been shown to have positive effects on immune function, blood sugar and ageing. It's been found that people who are self-compassionate are more likely to look after themselves and adopt healthy lifestyle habits. People who write themselves a self-compassionate letter every day for seven days are happier even three months later. In short, the links between self-compassion, health and happiness are overwhelming.

Self-compassion is the practice of extending kindness towards yourself. It's about being there for ourselves and empowering ourselves to alleviate our own suffering. If one of your close friends or a child was going through a difficult time, you wouldn't criticise them for not being good enough or judge them for any perceived shortcomings. You would offer them warmth, compassion and understanding. Sadly, many of us struggle to treat ourselves in the same way.

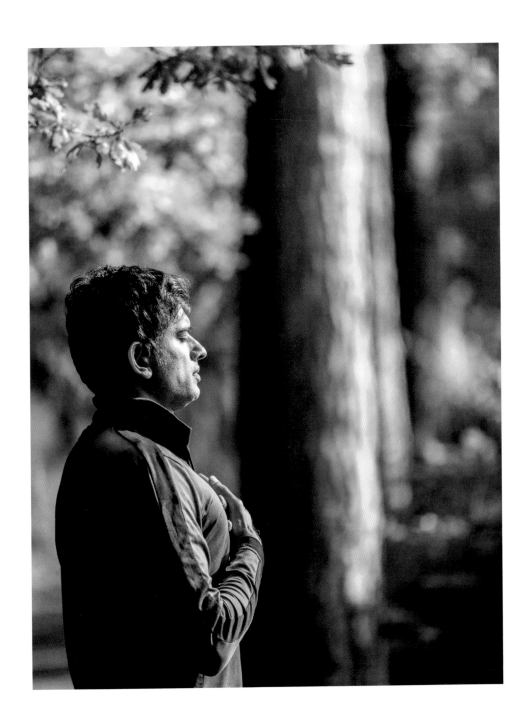

"

It's not possible to
achieve longtime
health or happiness
if you hate yourself.

"

THE SCIENCE OF SELF-TALK

Self-compassion starts in the mind, with the voice we hear in our heads. So many of us beat ourselves up in a way that's horribly abusive, just as I used to do. Multiple times a day, we talk to ourselves in ways we'd never dream of doing with our friends, our colleagues, or even complete strangers. Every time we speak to ourselves like this, we become our own worst enemies. We kick hard at every single leg of the Core Happiness stool. We make ourselves feel less content, less in control and shove ourselves deeply out of alignment.

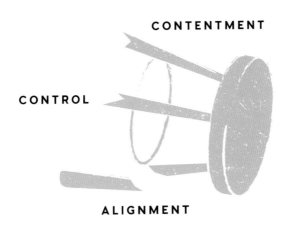

It's easy to think it doesn't really matter when we call ourselves a loser or an idiot. After all, nobody can hear us and it's only a brief flash of frustration that'll usually pass pretty quickly. But it's not trivial. When we do this, we're fighting with ourselves. The body responds as if we're in danger. Our stress response system gets activated. The biological effects of this activation are no less powerful than that of a prescription drug. Hormones such as adrenaline, noradrenaline and cortisol surge. We become hyper-vigilant and hyper-alert to what's going on around us. Our blood sugar rockets, and so does our blood pressure. Digestion and sex drive are turned down, meaning we're more likely to put on weight and suffer from libido problems. That self-loathing pill we've prescribed ourselves is a terrible poison.

The tone we should be aiming for instead is that of a supportive coach – one who fully accepts who we are but who wants to help us improve. Research by the psychologist Ethan Kross finds that when we're in the midst of a high-pressure situation we should speak to ourselves as we would our child, our best friend or a work colleague we admire. He even recommends that we refer to ourselves using our own names. When we do this, we create a distance between ourselves and the problem, and this makes us feel more in control. This is the opposite of what I was doing at the pool hall when I was a student. Yes, I was talking to myself like a coach – but an aggressive and abusive one. Even when I won, because of my underlying lack of self-worth, I didn't feel joy – I just felt relieved. And, if I lost, I'd feel awful after the game, and plug the hole I'd ripped in my heart by scoffing sugar, drinking or heading to the casino.

The psychologist Dr Pippa Grange, author of the wonderful book *Fear Less*, talks about this pattern of behaviour as 'winning shallow' versus 'winning deep'. I think this is a beautiful way of thinking about it. How will you choose to win in life? By feeling good about who you are after your victory – by being aligned with the person you really want to be? Or will you choose the ill rewards of emptiness and loathing?

 (To hear my conversation with Dr Ethan Kross about how to harness the power of the voice inside our heads, visit www.drchatterjee.com/173; and to hear me talk to the wonderful Dr Pippa Grange about how to 'win deep', visit www.drchatterjee.com/126.)

Happy Mind, Happy Life

Write Yourself a Love Letter

A really useful practice to help cultivate self-compassion is to write a letter to yourself. Some people find this a challenging exercise to do initially but it really is worth persevering. I have seen the transformative effects time and time again. Use the following as guidance to help you get started:

- In a journal or blank piece of paper, write down some of the qualities you love about yourself and what you have managed to achieve in life, despite all the problems you have faced. Write with a tone of compassion, warmth and forgiveness.

- If you struggle with this, imagine someone you really look up to. Imagine what your ideal parent might look like, or a teacher at school who had a positive impact on you. Now, imagine what they would say about you and write yourself a love letter from that perspective.

- If you find writing a letter too tricky to start with, try writing down five qualities you like about yourself. For example, I am honest, I am kind, I am always there for my friends, etc.

- Once you have the qualities written down, you could try expanding each one by writing a line or two about an example from your life where you demonstrated that quality.

I would recommend that you repeat this exercise regularly. Some of my patients practise this daily, but even once a week can have a powerful effect. And please don't be put off if you find it initially hard. The more you do it, the easier it becomes.

YOU ARE ENOUGH

Were you ever told that you were no good at something? Perhaps you were told that you were rubbish at playing the piano, or terrible at doing maths. Or perhaps you were told that you were no good at time-keeping and were always turning up late? The reality is that very few of us got through our childhoods without feeling as if we were being criticized for something or another, and that is exactly the moment when our inner critic is born. We internalized the criticism we received from others and then started using it against ourselves.

Your inner voice will try to criticize you first, before someone else has the opportunity to do so. It's important to understand that this is a protective mechanism that, as a child, helped you change your behaviour so that you could fit in with the world around you. As a child, your parents or carers are of crucial importance, as you rely on them for safety, shelter and survival. You will do whatever is required to fit in and keep the peace. Even if your parents were wonderful in a million different ways, there's every chance that from time to time you interpreted their actions and words in a way that made you feel as if you were not enough. And this core belief – that we are not enough – is responsible for a variety of troublesome adult traits such as jealousy, people-pleasing, insecurity and perfectionism.

Treating yourself with respect means understanding these childhood strategies for what they were and accepting that they no longer serve us. Instead, they keep us imprisoned and in mental turmoil. They're the core reason why so many of us just can't find it in us to love ourselves. We may not have felt unconditional love when our brains were developing and we were learning how to navigate the human world. We may have felt ignored, talked down to, at risk of being shouted at and punished. We may not have felt good enough in who we were to deserve kindness and love. And we never stop believing this. If we feel we're not good enough, we will

– often without knowing it – act in a way that manifests this belief. We self-sabotage our career opportunities and important relationships because, deep down, we think we don't deserve them. This is how not treating ourselves with respect can set major limits on our happiness.

The more we learn to treat ourselves with respect and compassion, the more we remind our brains that we are enough in who we are. As a consequence, there becomes less for the inner voice to criticize and, little by little, it starts to quieten and fade away.

CASE STUDY

Forty-eight-year-old Katherine was experiencing pain in her upper arms and abdomen. She felt bloated and was having trouble sleeping. Several doctors had run tests, but they had found nothing. They were puzzled. Katherine was fit and healthy, she'd improved her diet, taken up meditation, and had started going for a daily walk after dinner. But nothing seemed to help.

When she came to see me, I asked about her wider life. It turned out she had a history of romantic difficulties. She said she'd always end up with men who'd treat her badly. Sometimes, they were married, and it was typical for them to ghost her for weeks on end. 'Why does this always happen to me?' she asked.

As we talked, I started to suspect this underlying pattern had its roots in Katherine's childhood. She always felt her older sister got more attention than she did. She'd learned to accept having less attention bestowed on her than she wanted. This was once her strategy for survival, and she hadn't unlearned this in adulthood. Ultimately, her problem was that she didn't feel she was enough.

It took about eighteen months, but after practising self-compassion exercises several times a week, Katherine found herself in a stable relationship with a man of her age who was decent to her. She told me that, for the first time in her life, she felt like an equal. Shortly after the start of the relationship, her symptoms had pretty much resolved.

ARE YOU AN ADDICT?

We all have a hole in our hearts that, in moments of strife, we seek to fill with Junk Happiness. For some, the go-to is sugar. For others it's shopping, gaming, punishing sessions in the gym or drugs. Many fill the hole in their hearts with work. They're often the kind of people who might treat those they see as 'addicts' with pity and even a hint of contempt. But they don't realize that they're no less addicted: it's just that their compulsion has been deemed 'OK' by society, because it serves the Want Brain world.

It's probably fair to say that I've spent much of my life addicted to parts of my work. I used to believe that achievement would make me truly happy. In one of the podcast conversations I've had with him, the wonderful Dr Gabor Maté told me: 'There's a part of you that still believes that in order to validate your existence, you've got to put pressure on yourself to do more than your body can bear.' He was absolutely right. So while I understand the work-addict mindset, I also know the problems it brings. It means our self-respect is based on external metrics of success. This is ruinous for our Core Happiness because it means we're completely out of control. If you're a CEO and your self-worth is dependent on the value of your company, what happens if the stock market crashes and your business folds? Similarly, if all your identity is wrapped up in being a model parent, what happens when your child screams at you that they hate you? Usually, we compensate with even more Junk Happiness.

But here's the amazing thing about self-compassion: it actually makes people more successful. It helps us smash through the ceilings we've set for ourselves. When we know who we are and cease being scared of failure, we start to live a life without the limitations we've set for ourselves. Psychologists find that students who were taught to be more self-compassionate about failure ended up studying more. Contrary to the prevailing belief, self-compassion is associated with higher, not lower, motivation: if we're kind to ourselves, and feel less fear of failure, we go further.

We also embrace more of what life has to offer. I've noticed this over the past few years, as I've been working on my Core Happiness. I used to only play sports I excelled at. I didn't want to put myself in a position where I could fail, because I'd find that too painful. Now, I'll have a great time playing anything with my mates. I'm still competitive, but it has a different flavour. Whether I win or lose, I know this has no connection with my self-worth. If I lose, that's fine, because everyone loses at times. If I win, I also don't feel that superficial, artificial elevation that I once did. I won a game. That's all. No more, no less. My victory is not a reflection of who I am.

 (To hear the podcast conversations I had with Dr Gabor Maté about addiction, visit drchatterjee. com/37 and drchatterjee.com/169.)

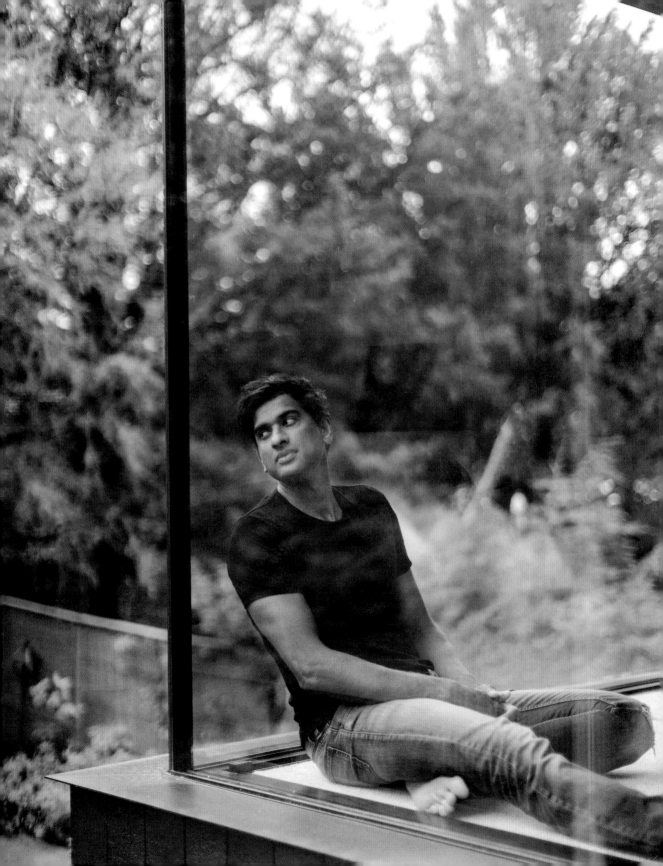

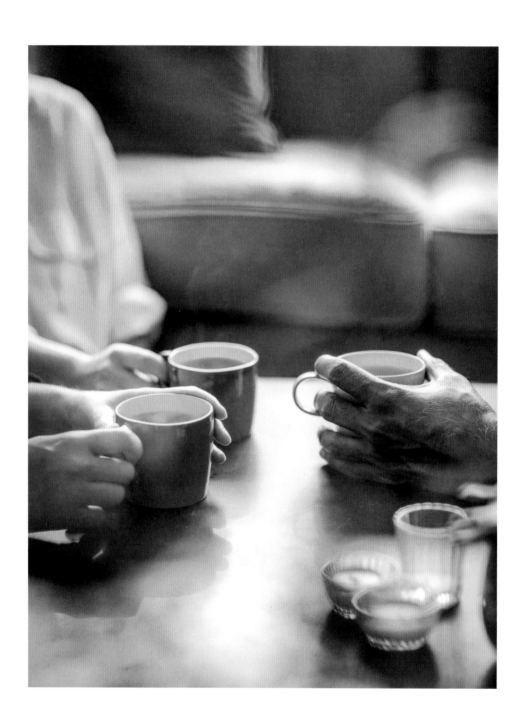

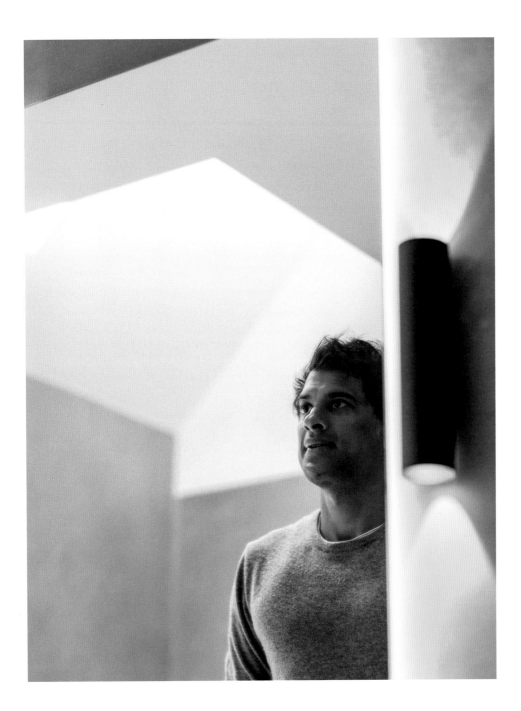

CASE STUDY

A couple of years ago I started seeing 52-year-old Pamela as a patient. She was overweight and generally unhealthy and was in a state of despair at her inability to stick to any new health regime. Her diet plans and New Year's resolutions would be successful for a few weeks, even sometimes a couple of months, but the weight would always come back. The same went for her attempts at starting regular exercise. She'd buy an online yoga class and give up after three sessions.

I got a hint of what the problem was when she came in to see me on a beautiful bright spring morning. 'Gorgeous day, isn't it?' I said as she walked in.

'Yeah, and how long is it going to last?' she replied.

I asked her to tell me what she typically says to herself, when she falls off any health plan she's trying her best to follow. 'I literally try to destroy myself in my head.' She tells herself that she's a failure, that she can't stick to anything, and that nothing ever works for her. She then goes on to binge on sugar and alcohol and spends hours online shopping to make herself feel better. The next day, she'll wake up feeling guilty, and the self-hatred starts up all over again.

I explained to her that her negative self-talk was making sustainable weight loss almost impossible. I asked her to catch herself whenever she said anything negative and try to reframe it as positive. I also asked her to start doing the mirror exercise five times a week. In common with many people who struggle with self-compassion, she found this extremely difficult. She worked up to it by writing down five qualities she liked about herself each day in a journal. After a couple of weeks, she was able to both write these down and then tell them to herself in the mirror.

When I saw her again six weeks later, there was a noticeable change in Pamela's demeanour. She seemed a lot more content and told me that her life felt less out of control. Her language was noticeably more positive and there was no doubt in my mind that she seemed a lot happier. She told me that she felt ready to start making small changes to her diet and lifestyle and was not interested any more in following punishing and gruelling health plans.

Over time, she began to lose weight slowly and sustainably. About six months after I first saw her, she was like a different person. She had lost a significant amount of weight in a way that she described as 'effortless'. She was also sleeping better, doing yoga regularly and prioritizing time for herself each day – she told me she's the happiest she's been since she was a little girl.

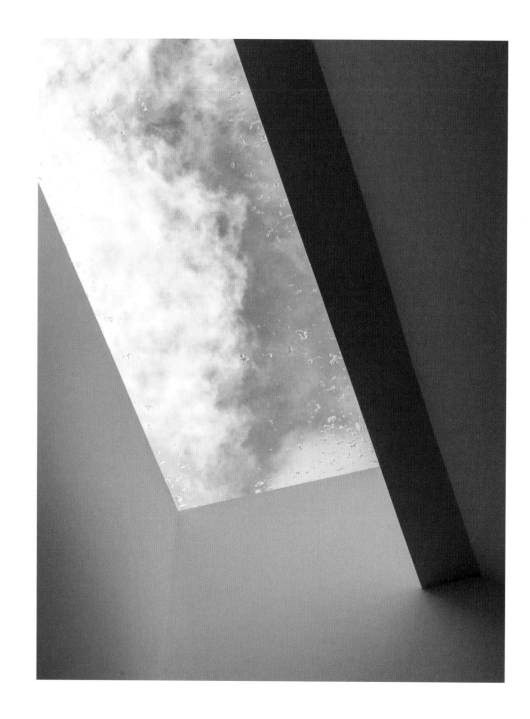

CONCLUSION

Having worked on self-compassion for several years, the voice I now hear in my head is exceptionally kind. I realize my competitiveness came from a place of not feeling enough in who I was, which in turn came from ideas I had formed in childhood. That belief served me when I was small. It helped me get the validation I was seeking from the world around me. But as an adult and a father, it was harming me by pushing me to do more than I could bear and was leading me towards the poisonous perils of Junk Happiness. These days, I love the person I see in the mirror, and I always feel good about myself, whether I win or lose. And this has had a huge impact on my life. Yes, I feel happier and more content, but I also find it much easier to stay engaged and be consistent with any lifestyle changes I am trying to make.

№ 4

MAKE TIME
STAND STILL

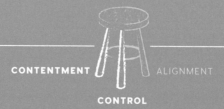

CONTENTMENT · ALIGNMENT

CONTROL

It's 8.30 p.m. on an ordinary Tuesday. The kitchen has been tidied and wiped, and you've just sat down on the sofa with a long sigh of relief. Finally, you have an hour or so to relax. You pick up your phone to check your notifications. There's a WhatsApp from your sister asking a question about your mum's upcoming birthday and an SMS from Yodel informing you about a package that is arriving tomorrow. No problem. You quickly reply to your sister, and authorize Yodel to leave the parcel on the back doorstep. Before you put the phone down, you check Twitter, then Instagram, leave a few likes and a cheeky comment for your cousin, then your partner comes in. You switch on the television, spend a few minutes flicking around: BBC, ITV, Netflix, Channel 5, Discovery. Your phone beeps. Your sister has replied to your WhatsApp. You thumb her an emoji. Another whizz past Instagram, Facebook and a glance at the news headlines. As you put your phone back down, you check the clock. It's 9.17 p.m. Where did all that time go?

NO TIME, NO HAPPINESS

The feeling of being 'time poor' has become an epidemic among adults. It's been found that an incredible 80 per cent of employed men and women feel this way, and most stay-at-home parents also report the same time poverty. But is it actually true? People are often surprised when I say this, but the research shows we actually have *more* leisure time than we did fifty years ago. If we don't feel that we do, it's often because the me-time we have these days is massively degraded. We're surrounded by modern technology that fragments and disrupts our time. How would we have spent those precious forty-seven minutes back in the 1970s? Listening to the radio while lost in a hobby, doing some ironing with your favourite album on in the background or, perhaps, watching one of the three programmes that was scheduled for 8.30 p.m, undistracted, with our partner. Up until very recently, most people had daily periods in which time slowed down and they could just be.

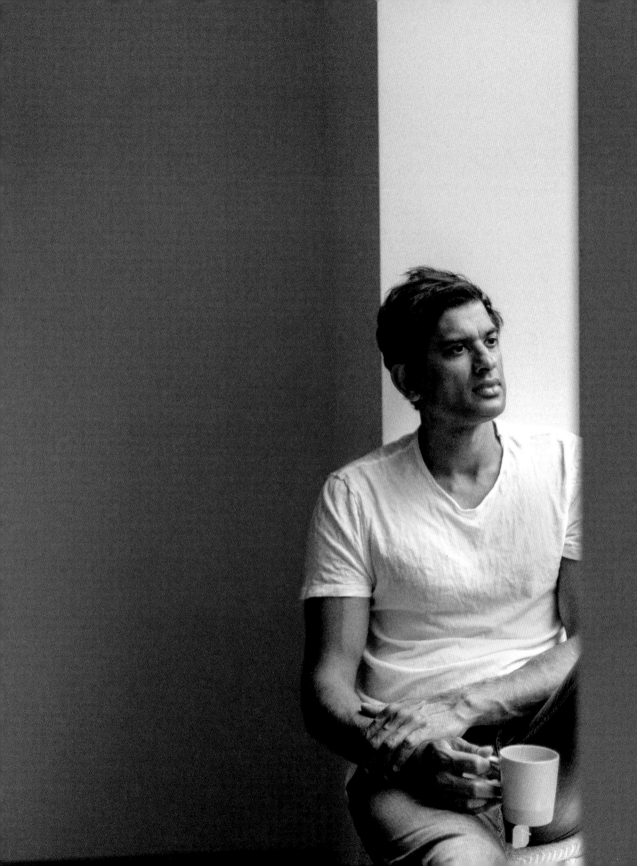

TIME IS LIFE

For me, thinking about 'time quality' was a true paradigm shift. My life changed for the better when I started seeing my time as something valuable that I owned and should protect and defend. It's no exaggeration to say that time is the most precious resource we have. The wonderful thing about it is that we all have the same amount of time each day as the wealthiest person on earth. But all too often, we don't treasure it. We waste it. We allow it to become diluted by using it mindlessly. Think of it like this. What is time? Time is life. Literally: the time you have is the life you have. And yet, every day, we allow this unimaginably precious resource to run through our fingers like water.

This problem is made worse by the Want Brain world we all live in. We're taught to admire people who are time poor. Being busy is seen as a status symbol. We associate it with being in demand and successful. To make matters worse, we're taught to value money more than time. We happily spend our leisure time trying to save every penny we can on every item we buy, searching online, comparing prices on different websites, trying to find the very best deal – and it never occurs to us that we're 'spending' our time as we do this. If you spend three hours online to make a £2 saving on a new camera or a new pair of shoes, is it worth it? Are we *really* getting the best deal when we behave this way? Sometimes we are, depending on our own individual circumstances. But, on many occasions, we won't be.

I am not saying that we should never be comparing prices. I am simply encouraging you to start thinking about your time account in the same way that you might think about your bank account. How you value your time will be different to how I value my time. We have different lives, different income levels and different priorities. That is completely OK. All of us need to do what is right for us. But, for many of us, we have never even asked ourselves the question: how valuable is our time?

The perception that we have enough time in our lives is essential for Core Happiness. Simply feeling that we have some space in our schedules for ourselves makes us feel more content and in control, directly strengthening two legs of the Core Happiness stool. We know that when working adults use money to buy themselves time as opposed to material goods, they are happier, and that people gain about 50 per cent of the happiness of getting married simply by valuing time more. And, importantly, this boost in happiness is also seen at lower income levels.

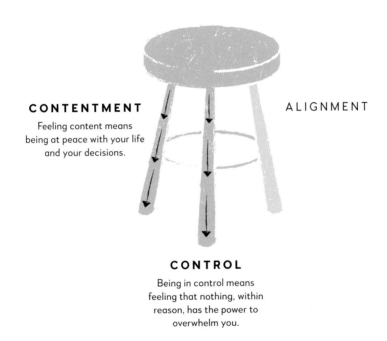

CONTENTMENT
Feeling content means
being at peace with your life
and your decisions.

ALIGNMENT

CONTROL
Being in control means
feeling that nothing, within
reason, has the power to
overwhelm you.

People often think that valuing time over money is something that only the wealthy have the luxury to think about. But this is simply not the case. Professor Ashley Whillans from the Harvard Business School studied a group of women in Kenya who earned around $10 a day. They worked full time, had kids at home and struggled to make ends meet. Whillans split them into two groups that received either a time saving or some extra money. Both the time and the money were equivalent to three days' worth of labour. One might have predicted that people living in poverty would gain greater benefits from receiving more money over a saving of time. However, both groups improved their wellbeing, reduced stress and increased their relationship satisfaction scores to the same degree. And, remarkably, the women who were given the time saving had longer-lasting positive effects. So even in these harsh conditions of poverty and struggle, valuing time over money has a positive effect on happiness.

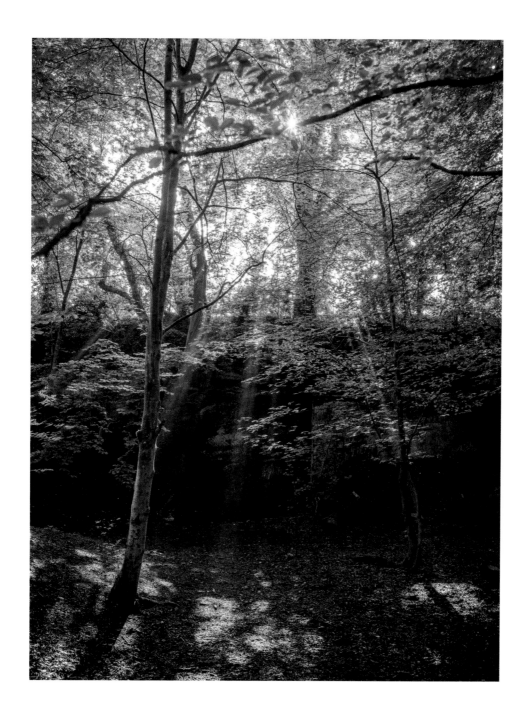

MORE TIME, BETTER HEALTH

People who feel time poor are more stressed, less productive and less happy in their lives. They're also more likely to engage in more unhealthy behaviours: they eat more high-calorie food, exercise less and are at higher risk of suffering from a chronic disease. They're also more anxious and depressed. Professor Ashley Whillans finds experiencing 'time famine' can be as bad for our mental health as being unemployed for an entire year. She believes the secret to happiness is prioritizing 'time over money – one decision at a time'.

This research echoes what I've seen over and over again with my patients. People who feel they don't have time are much less likely to engage in healthy lifestyle habits, such as exercise or cooking good meals from scratch. Their background stress levels are also elevated, which further impacts all kinds of symptoms, including migraines, gut problems, anxiety, mood issues and hormonal issues. Time famine can also play havoc with sleep. Not only do people who feel they don't have time find it harder to switch off and fall asleep, they stay up later, as they feel a need to 'unwind', often with the help of wine and perhaps endless social media scrolling. Often, simply solving the upstream problem of feeling deprived of time has amazing downstream impacts on physical health.

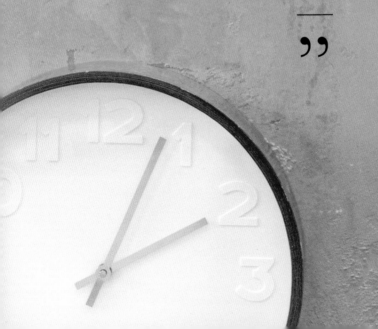

"

The time you have
is the life you have.

"

CASE STUDY

One of my patients, 55-year-old Tim, would come in to see me regularly with a variety of stress-related symptoms like insomnia, fatigue and anxiety. This was having a negative impact on his close relationships. He also had a background frustration that he was always looked over for promotions at work.

He didn't earn much money and was always counting the pennies, trying to find the best deal. Whenever he came to see me in my consultation room he would make it clear to me that he didn't have time to focus on his health. Money was tight and that was where he had to put his energy.

When I looked into his life to see how I might help him make some changes, two things he did each week to save money jumped out at me. Once a week, he would drive fifteen minutes out of town to get cheaper petrol, and he would also visit three different shops on multiple occasions to get the best deals on the food he was buying for his family.

When we looked at these situations in detail, we worked out that each week he was saving around two pence per litre on a thirty-litre refuel – this was a sixty-pence saving for thirty minutes of his time. He was saving a little bit more money with his visit to three different food stores – about £8 per week – but it was costing him an extra two hours of his time, compared to going to just one.

I explained to him that, effectively, he was using up two and a half hours of his weekly time to 'earn' £8.60. I asked him to imagine what he might be able to do each week with an extra 150 minutes. For the first time in his life, he had started to put an actual value on the worth of his free time.

After reflecting, he could see that he was 'spending' the equivalent of twenty-five minutes a day to save £8.60 each week. He initially felt uneasy about giving up the money saving, but we managed to agree on a short experiment. For the next four weeks he would fill up with petrol at the nearest fuel station and do all of his household shopping in his local supermarket, once a week. In the time that he saved, he would do something proactive for his health.

With this extra time, he began to take a daily walk and started to feel less time poor. This was not just coming from the time saving itself. Not driving through traffic and having to queue up three times in three different shops dramatically reduced his stress levels. And this started a ripple effect into other areas of his life. He felt as if he had more time to play with his kids and more time to unwind from work. This in turn made him feel calmer, the quality of his sleep improved and he felt closer and more connected with his wife.

Over the next few months, he started to prioritize time in other areas of his life. Within a year, he had not only got a promotion at work, he had also lost a stone in weight and his blood health markers had significantly improved. And he felt much happier. It all started with giving up £8.60 per week, in exchange for twenty-five minutes a day.

Time versus Money

I would like you to perform an audit on your own life to see when you are valuing money over time. Of course, this exercise will depend on your own financial circumstances and the dynamics of your own life. Are there any instances where you might be able to make a different trade-off and prioritize your time more?

Here are some common scenarios to get you thinking:

- Do you spend hours researching the best deal for a new product online? How much money do you really save? What might you be able to do with that time instead?

- How many times do you go to the supermarket each week? What is the time cost each time? If you drive, what is the fuel cost? What if you went only once a week or ordered an online shop to come at the same time each week? How might that impact the quality of your life?

- How much do you spend on coffee out each week? Make sure you factor in the time it takes you to get to the coffee shop as well as the price of the coffee. Would a home coffee machine help? Of course, there are other benefits from going to a coffee shop, like interacting with others, and so on. This is simply about asking yourself to review and see if you might be better off making a different choice. Over the course of a few months, you are likely to save time and money with a home coffee machine. What could you do with that extra time? Would it be worth it for you?

- When going on holiday, do you try to book every single aspect of the holiday yourself? The flight, the hotel, the car hire, the transfers, and so on. How much extra would it really cost to have a travel agent do it for you? Would it be worth it for you to pay a little bit more for your holiday but massively reduce the stress?

- Are you able to sacrifice some of your income in order to have more help at home; for example, cleaners or childcare? What would that extra time bring to your life?

- Do you enjoy cooking fresh, wholesome meals but find buying all the ingredients needed and the right recipe time-consuming and stress-inducing? Perhaps a meals service where they deliver you all the fresh ingredients, pre-chopped and in the right amounts, along with an easy-to-follow recipe card might help you enjoy more time, even though it will probably cost a little bit more.

Over time, once you have become aware, it becomes easier to start valuing time over money. And when we do – within our own means – we experience less stress, have stronger social relationships and feel happier overall.

TIME IS FLUID

And here's the great news: we can create the perception of having more time, even if we don't. Of course, one day will always be twenty-four hours long, just as sixty minutes will always add up to one hour, and there's nothing anyone can do to change that. But one hour watching paint dry is experienced in a completely different way to one hour hanging out with a close friend. When it comes to time, the mind truly does have power over matter. Our perception of time changes its reality. We can control it, and become time affluent by making the clock stand still.

The first step is making sure we're using our time intentionally. Rather than letting our me-time slip away without a thought, we can value it, plan it, defend it and then stretch it, getting more time out of those same sixty minutes. One of my own favourite methods of stretching time is playing snooker. For sure, I enjoy playing with my children, but I also deeply love playing snooker by myself. When I'm alone, there's no one to impress. There's no showboating. I don't post about it on social media afterwards. I do it purely for the intrinsic pleasure of the game. I become hypnotized by it. I love the sound of the balls clacking together. I love thinking about the different angles, how the spin has different effects depending on how and where I hit the white ball. I could be playing for ten minutes or an hour – I honestly have no real idea, because I'm mesmerized. The clock doesn't stand still as much as vanish altogether. I'm not thinking about my work, I'm not thinking about my family, I'm not thinking about my life. I'm simply engrossed.

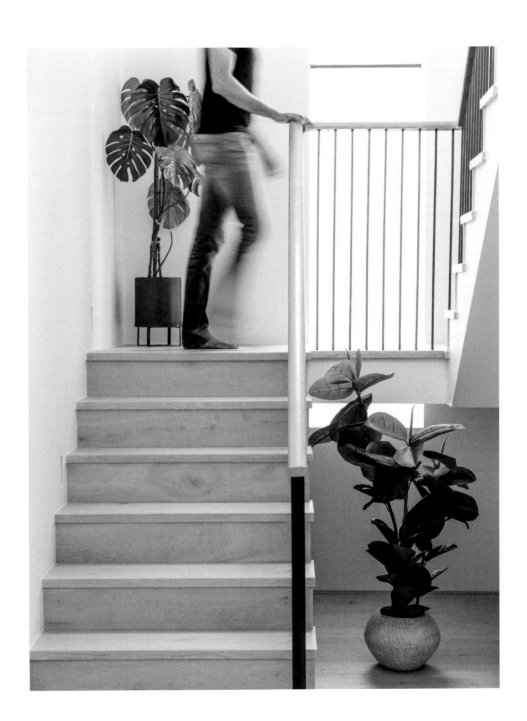

GET INTO THE FLOW

So what exactly is going on when I'm playing snooker and creating the sensation of time disappearing? I've entered an amazing frame of mind known as the 'flow state'. The term 'flow' was coined by the late psychologist Professor Mihaly Csikszentmihalyi. His research has shown that the more often people experience it, the greater their sense of wellbeing and life satisfaction. Flow has been shown to make people up to 500 per cent more productive, 600 per cent more creative and increase their thinking power so much it can cut learning times in half. If all that wasn't enough, flow can even make us more empathetic.

When we're in flow, we're literally in the moment. We're not ruminating about the past or tying ourselves up in knots about the future. As Csikszentmihalyi himself puts it, 'One of the most frequently mentioned dimensions of the flow experience is that, while it lasts, one is able to forget all the unpleasant aspects of life.' It powerfully activates all three legs of the Core Happiness stool simultaneously. When we're in flow, we feel utterly content, completely in control of the world, and are perfectly aligned inside and out: our thoughts and actions are one and the same. We're so focused on what we're doing, we feel as if we've 'left' our bodies.

If this is now sounding to you like a drug-induced experience, you're not far wrong. You might not realize it, but the brain is a chemical factory. Part of the reason that recreational drugs make people feel so good is because they release or mimic natural neurochemicals in large amounts. When we're in flow state, we're releasing a wonderful cocktail of these pleasure chemicals. No less than five of our most powerful neurochemicals start to surge: dopamine, the so-called 'reward' chemical; norepinephrine, which helps drive focus, excitement and attention; anandamide, which helps reduce pain and stress while ramping up our creative powers; endorphins, which are the body's own version of heroin, and also reduce stress and pain; and, finally, serotonin, which calms us at the end of a flow state.

No wonder scientists believe flow to be the most addictive natural feeling there is.

The surest way to trigger these pleasure chemicals, and enter flow, is to try learning or mastering an activity that you love. I fall most deeply into flow when I'm trying to learn a new snooker shot, or working on a new idea for a song on my guitar. The challenge your task presents should be just a little bit harder than your current skill set allows. If it is too easy, you'll get bored and your mind will wander. If it's too difficult, you'll become frustrated. The best research suggests that, for most of us, the challenge of the task should be around 4 per cent higher than our skill level. Of course, I'm not expecting you to measure this. Simply use that idea as a guide. When we hit that sweet spot, we enter what's called the 'flow channel'.

Psychologists describe flow as having six core components:

1. Complete concentration on the task in hand. Our thoughts and actions become one.

2. The sense of self decreases; the ego is quietened.

3. Our perception of time changes.

4. The sense of anxious struggle disappears.

5. The sense of control increases. The task provides immediate feedback, which helps psychological immersion.

6. The task becomes a pleasurable experience in and of itself.

 (To hear more about the benefits of flow and how to access it more easily, you can listen to a podcast conversation I had with Steven Kotler, an expert in flow, at www.drchatterjee.com/189.)

FLOW FOLLOWS FOCUS

My friend and running coach Helen Hall gets into 'flow' when she is trying to learn a new skill – subtly changing the position of her pelvis when she runs, for example. She's looking for mastery, and this increased focus helps slip her into flow state. People like Helen are lucky enough to access flow regularly at work. And many of us do, especially in creative professions; for example, architects, writers and painters. I myself can enter flow when I am recording a long podcast conversation with someone I deeply respect and admire, or when I am writing. If you're in a job that doesn't put you into a flow state, that is completely fine. Simply try to find ways of accessing flow state in your own time.

These kinds of activities are very often creative, and can involve building things. The furniture maker Gary Rogowski writes, 'People have the need to put their hands on tools and to make things. We need this in order to feel whole. Long ago we learned to think by using our hands, not the other way round.' To create is to be human, but we're too often engaged in jobs that don't result in any obvious tangible result that we can see or touch. You might not think of yourself as a creative person, but I believe there's no such thing as a non-creative human. So what can you create? Will you put up a shelf, paint a room, or write a poem, a story or a song? Remember, you're not competing with anyone. This isn't about ambition, it's about triggering your focus and moving into flow.

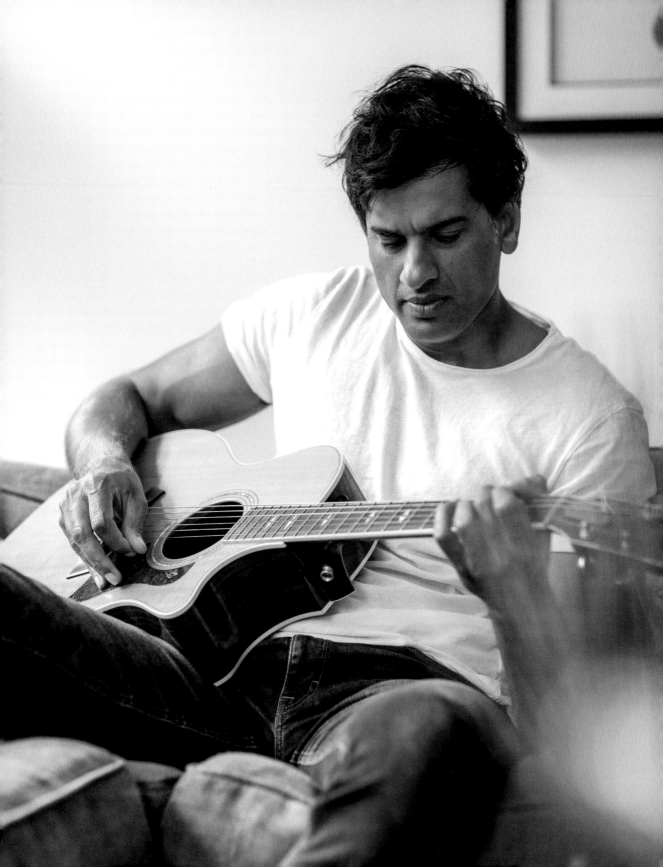

Finding Your Flow

There are infinite ways to access flow state. I would like you to find something that works for you at your current stage in life. If you are not sure where to start, think about the things you used to love as a child, like playing the piano, drawing, painting or building Lego. Don't feel self-conscious about these hobbies, as if they're things that might be considered childish. Play is a crucial ingredient for health and wellbeing and we often forget that as we get older. We're simply looking for activities that you can immerse yourself in, which you enjoy and find challenging, and where time starts to stand still.

Here are some examples of people accessing flow state to get you thinking:

- A pool player trying to learn a trick shot

- A graphic designer coming up with a new logo

- A teacher coming up with a new way of communicating an idea

- A game of tennis where your opponent is just a little bit better than you

- Solving a Rubik's cube

- A writer when 'in the zone'

- A musician 'in the slot'

- A cook creating a complex meal

- A mountain biker trying to navigate a downhill route

- A runner running through a forest with multiple obstacles

- A DIY enthusiast trying to put up a shelf in their shed

If there's nothing you can think of that you can practise and get lost in alone, why not join a club or organize a regular activity with friends? I know a guy who used to love playing Xbox with his mates. Now gaming has moved online, he misses the social connection, and the banter, chat and camaraderie that would've built up between games. He made a point of asking his three best friends to commit to one evening a week where they could meet and play in person. Needless to say, all three of them are far happier now that they're getting their regular sessions of connection and flow.

Aim to access flow state at least one to two times each week. Flow state is when we feel most alive. Regularly accessing flow will make it easier to get through busy days, helps reduce the likelihood of burnout and helps us experience more joy.

CONCLUSION

Feeling constantly short of time damages Core Happiness and health. But even the busiest among us can change our experience of time, making it feel as if we have more. It's simply a matter of finding something that we're passionate about and that fully absorbs us. Even twenty minutes twice a week will make a big difference. So what will you do? How will you change your life by spending just a bit of time doing something you love?

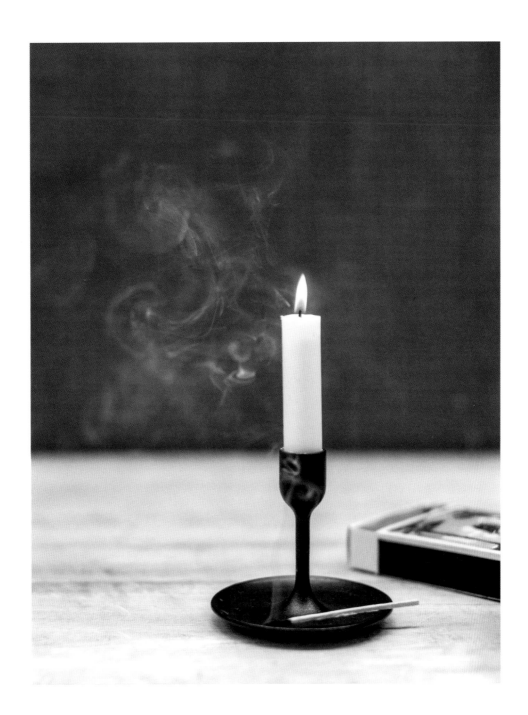

№ 5

SEEK OUT FRICTION

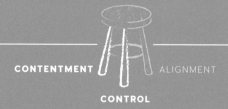

CONTENTMENT — ALIGNMENT

CONTROL

We think of a happy life as one in which everything goes our way. If happiness is our ultimate goal, then surely a life free from stresses, strains and friction is what we should be aiming for? However, this is an impossible goal. We might experience short spells of perfect calm very occasionally, but the reality of life is that you're continually being presented with new challenges. No amount of practice or planning can prevent new issues popping up all over your well-tended life like stubborn weeds.

To build Core Happiness, we can make our problems work for us, not against us. And there's one particular kind of problem that I've found to be especially useful for building happiness. Because humans are highly social creatures, many of the issues we encounter day to day inevitably involve other people. We all exist in a web of humanity, whether it's family, colleagues or members of our communities. This simple fact brings with it inevitable challenges. I don't need to tell you that humans (ourselves included!) can be complex and unpredictable. Often, our interactions with others can leave us feeling angry, frustrated and disappointed. But if we learn to look at the same situation through different eyes, social friction can actually be a major source of strength.

THE SOCIAL GYM

Just as our muscles grow when they experience regular resistance, so our Core Happiness becomes stronger when we press up against other people. But this can only happen when we tackle social tension in a very specific way. I think of it as using the human world as a social gym. This means seeking out moments of friction and using them as ways to examine ourselves. If someone says something that makes me react badly, I have two choices. I can get frustrated, worked up and make myself a victim. I can tell myself a story that the other person was rude, out of order and should not have behaved in this manner. If they had acted differently, my world would be much better. This is how most people react. But there is an alternative – you can make the choice to use friction as a teacher by asking yourself, 'Why is this comment triggering me? What is it inside me that's causing me to react in this way?'

When we do this, we take back control over our life and feel more content, immediately strengthening two legs of the Core Happiness stool. We are no longer dependent on everyone around us acting in a certain way in order for us to be happy. By using the world as a social gym, we give ourselves the opportunity to become stronger multiple times a day. I've been practising this technique for the last three years or so, and it's no exaggeration to say that, as a result, I now feel pretty bulletproof. Whereas I used to sometimes get triggered when someone, for example, made a negative comment about me on social media, I now use these comments as an opportunity to learn more about myself.

If you're truly secure and happy, the things other people say won't bother you. If you're regularly analysing all the criticism you get, in a calm way, then criticism that's fair won't have the power to knock you off your feet. It will simply cause you to reflect and perhaps modify your opinion or actions. And if it's unfair? Then you can swat it away with ease. The same is true of praise. Flattery can't go to your head and distort your thinking when your sense of who you are is based on regular, calm analysis of social friction. I honestly don't mind having a day that includes ten bits of friction, as long as I respond to them in a healthy way. I view it as free therapy. My trolls come bearing gifts.

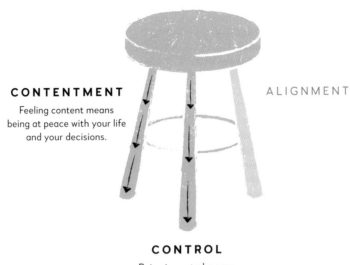

CONTENTMENT

Feeling content means being at peace with your life and your decisions.

ALIGNMENT

CONTROL

Being in control means feeling that nothing, within reason, has the power to overwhelm you.

When you're dependent on other people interacting with you in a certain way, you make yourself their prisoner. Seeking out friction allows you to become a master of your own happiness. When you practise using friction as a teacher, bit by bit, you start to change. You become less reactive and more content in yourself. Triggering social moments become much less powerful. You're able to create extra space between the frictional event and your reaction to it. This can feel hard in the moment, and it certainly takes practice. But in six months' time, you'll be transformed.

MAKE EVERYONE A HERO

The psychologist Dr Edith Eger knows more than most about how to deal with life's frictions. When she was a teenager living in Nazi-occupied Eastern Europe she was sent to the Auschwitz death camp with her parents. Her mother and father were murdered in the gas chamber the day they got there, but Edith survived. She was rescued in 1945 by an American soldier who, by sheer luck, saw her hand twitch in a pile of corpses. When I spoke to her on my podcast, she was ninety-three years old and she looked back on that time with an incredible and powerful spirit of deep forgiveness. She told me that, in Auschwitz, she didn't consider herself a prisoner of the Nazis. Instead, she reframed the situation in her mind, so that the guards became the prisoners. In Edith's imagination, she was entirely free. She told me, 'The greatest prison you'll ever live in is the prison you create inside your mind.'

I think about those words every day. Just as Edith managed to do in the absolute hell of Auschwitz, we can actively decide how to frame the world. If we choose to, we can tell ourselves a negative story about our lives that says, 'I am a victim.' We can tell ourselves, 'This always happens to me,' and blame all our personal failures on other people. Or we can consciously change the story. We can walk around to the other side of our reality and see it from a different, more positive perspective.

My conversation with Edith taught me that when we see ourselves as a victim, we become our own victimizer. Of course, I do not wish to downplay the serious events that sometimes happen in life where it is really hard to not see yourself as a victim. However, many of us have an inner tendency to want to see ourselves as one, even when the fault's actually with us. This is human nature. Everyone lets themselves off the hook this way, to some extent. But victim-mindedness is terrible for our mental wellbeing. It weakens our Core Happiness by making us feel less content with the world and less in control. When we work to change our inner story, consciously taking ourselves out of the victim role, we become empowered.

We become less reactive, more confident and more in command of our lives.

One powerful technique for achieving this involves reframing our inner story so that everyone we react to negatively, in our day-to-day lives, becomes a hero. As you might remember, during the early weeks of the 2020 Covid pandemic, there was a national toilet-roll shortage. Everyone got used to turning up to the supermarket to find the shelves empty, then switching on the news at home to see people staggering to their cars with trollies loaded with huge multipacks of three-ply. It was the easiest thing in the world to see these people as villains, and ourselves as their victims.

But we could also walk around to the other side of that story and see it from a different direction. Did they, perhaps, work in a care home? Maybe they looked after four elderly grandparents who were incontinent? Or were they planning to sell their hoard on eBay for a fat profit? If so, do you view these people as selfish, or could it be that they are struggling for cash and, in their minds, this seems like a reasonable way to make some money to feed their families? Or perhaps they were the exception and the empty shelves were actually the result of hundreds of perfectly reasonable people thinking, 'I'll buy one extra pack, just in case.'

The point is, when it comes to our happiness, it doesn't matter which story is true. All that matters is how we feel about it. There are infinite situations we will face in the world that we cannot change. But we *can* change our reaction. We create our own reality. By making these people a hero, we win. We become kinder, calmer, less judgemental, easier to be around – and a lot happier.

 (To listen to an incredible conversation I had with Edith Eger on my podcast, go to www.drchatterjee. com/144.)

CHOOSE YOUR STORY

It's all too easy to fall into the trap of becoming so sure of our view of the world that we forget we're only seeing it from one narrow perspective. Psychologists have been studying these effects for years. In one experiment, they looked at how different sets of football fans judged the same piece of match footage. When they watched the video of the game and were then asked what happened in it, they reported seeing different things. This is how we live our lives. What about when a couple have a disagreement? Both sides have their own version of what happened. They each tell themselves their own story and, in their own heads, they know the 'truth'. Each one is their truth, but which 'truth' is right? Neither. The reality of these incidents is that they're always subjective. We all write our own truth. So why not choose a truth that makes us happier?

If you have any doubt about the life-changing possibilities of reframing your world, consider the case of John McAvoy. He grew up surrounded by criminals and became an armed robber, finally being arrested in 2005 after a failed attempt at stealing £100,000 from a security van. When he was in prison, he saw footage of a police chase in the Netherlands in which one of his best friends had been killed. It forced him to reassess the story he told about the world which said he was a victim of 'the system'. He made the positive decision to take responsibility for his thefts and for traumatizing innocent bank workers. Having accepted that his whole life had been based on a lie, he empowered himself by telling a new story. At that time, he was overweight, serving a life sentence in prison, but he decided to start rowing. This changed his life. While still in prison, he broke three world and seven British records for rowing. He has since been released and is now a world-famous triathlete, inspiring millions around the world. He is now giving back to society and speaks regularly to prisoners and schoolkids, inspiring them to live better lives. It all started with him consciously choosing to tell himself a new story. You can do the same too.

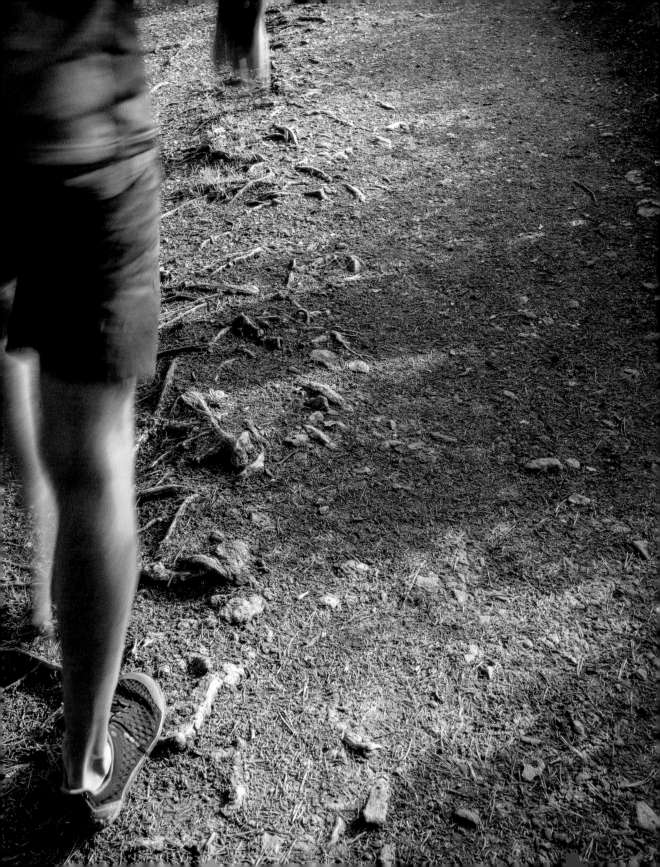

Working Out at the Social Gym

Over the course of one week, experiment with analysing a moment of social friction each day. This exercise need not take longer than five to ten minutes. The more you do it, the easier it gets, as you will be training yourself to take a different perspective on life's inevitable challenges.

At the end of the week, spend a few moments reflecting on how this exercise has made you feel. Do you feel calmer, more in control and more content? Are you sleeping better or feeling less anxious?

You are free to continue doing this every day, of course, if you would like. I would highly recommend you return to this exercise every time you find your happiness being negatively affected by somebody else. When you work out regularly in the social gym, life becomes significantly easier.

- When did I get triggered today? This could be a time when you felt frustrated, angry, annoyed or disappointed. It could also be when you fell into the trap of judging others.

- What was the reason? Was it because you didn't sleep well and reacted emotionally? Or was it because it highlighted your insecurities and reminded you of something in your past?

- What emotion did it bring up inside you? If you can, write down the emotions you felt.

- Try to feel where you feel that emotion in your body. See if you can breathe into that area and help the tension or tightness ease off.

- Reflect and think about or write down what this bit of friction has taught you about yourself. For example, 'I am not sleeping well at the moment, which is why I am overly emotional.' Or 'This situation has highlighted my inner insecurities about who I am. This is not about the other person, this is about me.'

- Now write a happiness story about the same situation but change your perspective to give you a sense of control over the situation. A useful tip here is to try to make the person you are thinking about a hero in some way.

- Try to feel compassion for them. Understand that they are probably taking out their own stresses and insecurities on you. In reality, their actions have nothing to do with you. You cannot influence them and, if you are waiting for other people to act in a certain way, in order for you to be happy, you will be waiting a very long time.

FRICTION LEADS TO COMPASSION

After nearly three hours talking to John McAvoy on my podcast I realized that, if I had had his upbringing, I'd probably have ended up in prison as well. This led me to think about how often we judge people and criticize their life decisions. We reflexively think, 'I can't believe they did that,' or 'What a stupid man!' The problem with this kind of thinking is that we all have a skewed view of the world and see it through our own unique lens. We don't often acknowledge how much we've been influenced by our own environments. If you grew up with hardly any money and very little opportunity in and outside school, you'd probably see the world through a different lens compared to someone who grew up in middle-class suburbia and had a private-school education. If your mother or father made themselves a victim whenever anything bad happened and said things like 'This always happens to me' or 'I can't believe they acted like that,' it's no surprise that you'll have similar tendencies.

Understanding that every one of us is a complex result of all our previous interactions and experience helps us develop a deep sense of empathy and compassion. It also helps us feel that the world is more predictable because we now understand why someone may have a different perspective. This helps build our sense of control, which is one leg of the Core Happiness stool.

A turning point in my life and levels of happiness came when I realized that everyone is doing the best they can, based upon their upbringing, knowledge and life situation. This was really brought home for me in a powerful conversation I had on my podcast with the writer and speaker Peter Crone. If you were the other person, with their childhood, their parents and their *exact* same life experiences, you would almost certainly be acting in exactly the same way. Our ego doesn't want to believe this. We tell ourselves that, if we were them, we'd behave differently. Because we're better than them and more knowledgeable and kinder. But this is just our ego talking. How could it be true? If they *could* act differently, they would. Understanding this has brought a new level of calm and perspective to my life. It makes it easier to be compassionate to every person I meet.

Choose the story that makes you happy,
not the one that holds you hostage.

 (To hear the inspirational life story of John McAvoy, and an incredible conversation I had with him on my podcast, visit www.drchatterjee.com/91. And, to learn more about how to change the story inside your mind, I'd highly recommend you listen to the powerful conversations I had with Peter Crone, a thought leader in human potential, by visiting www.drchatterjee.com/petercrone.)

How to be Less Judgemental

Humans can be incredibly judgemental about others. In most cases, the root cause is a feeling of inadequacy and not feeling good enough in ourselves. On other occasions, it comes more from jealousy, which itself tends to come from a fear of not being truly loveable for who we are. We try to make ourselves feel better by looking down on others.

In the short term, you may feel better – just like when we engage in many Junk Happiness habits – but, in the long term, judging others is highly problematic for your Core Happiness. It aggressively attacks all three legs of the Core Happiness stool – you feel less in control, less content with life and less aligned – as no one really wants to be the kind of person who looks down on others. Holding on to judgement of others keeps that version of them alive in your mind and this will slowly burn away at your inner happiness like acid.

The next time you find yourself judging someone else for what they have done or how they have acted, try to see if you can make them a hero.

Use the following questions to help you:

- Is the way I feel about that other person really true?

- Why is this situation really bothering me?

- How would it feel if I chose a different perspective?

- What's stopping me from making them a hero and choosing a story that empowers me rather than enslaves me?

What story could you write about them in your mind that would make the way they acted seem reasonable? Perhaps you could think about their upbringing and the pressures they have faced in their life. Perhaps they are going through a tough time at the moment. Could they or someone else close to them be suffering with a chronic disease, and that is causing them to act in the way that they are? Are they scared and feeling afraid about the future because their job is under threat? Or could it be that they have a young child who is up several times a night and it is leaving them exhausted and emotionally fragile?

The reality of the situation doesn't actually matter for your Core Happiness. All that matters is the story you choose to tell yourself. Don't choose a story that makes you a victim. Choose a story that empowers you and helps you feel calm and in control of the situation.

With time, this exercise will help you judge others less. It will help you to become more compassionate and forgiving. And, I guarantee, it will have a profound impact on your own levels of Core Happiness, as it already has on mine.

RISKING FRICTION

When I first went through the process of going through the Identity Menu (see page 39), I realized that 'integrity' is an extremely important value for me. In order to feel more aligned, and build Core Happiness, I needed to practise it as much as possible. A couple of years ago, I was asked to take part in an online event in August. At the time, I was completely slammed with work commitments. I felt really burned out and, two weeks before the request, I had made a promise to myself that I wasn't going to take on any new work commitments until after the summer. The only reason I even considered doing the event in the first place was because I really liked the organizer and did not want to let her down.

It would've been so easy to tell a white lie and say I was already booked, and the old me would have definitely taken that approach in my desire not to offend. But the new, empowered me who had taken time to truly understand his values knew I'd feel bad about it afterwards. That small moment of dishonesty would knock me out of alignment, and I'd be left with a nagging feeling I'd behaved dishonourably to someone I really like. Instead, I made the decision to risk a bit of social friction. I didn't take the easy route out by replying by text or email but instead phoned the organizer. I told her, 'I would dearly love to help you, but I've decided I'm not taking on any work commitments until September. I've got a couple of projects to finish off and then I'm spending the rest of the summer with my wife and kids.'

I was a little apprehensive about telling her the truth in case she thought less of me afterwards – a hangover from my people-pleasing days. To my surprise and relief, she was utterly lovely about it and completely understood. This helped me realize that the more you risk friction by telling your truth, the more aligned you become. It's true that this kind of social interaction can make you anxious in the short term, but it's undoubtedly a long-term win. And the more you do it, the easier it becomes.

"

Seeking out friction
allows you to become
a master of your
own happiness.

"

CASE STUDY

One of my patients, Brian, was an only child. At forty-seven, he began caring for his elderly mother. Brian was married with two children and had many competing demands on his time. With his responsibilities at home, at work and with his mother piling up, he started experiencing a lot of stress and anger, which affected his sleep and his marriage. He'd come to see me because, for the first time in his life, he'd started suffering from migraines.

Brian was made particularly irritable by the fact that his mother would call him up at any time of the day to come round and do little things: heat up dinner in the microwave, find the remote control, help her look for a jigsaw piece that she'd dropped. Sometimes he'd say to himself, 'If she really loved me, she wouldn't be acting like this.' He kept repeating this story to himself. He convinced himself this was true and that his mother didn't really care about him. This made him even more wound up.

I helped Brian use this social friction as an opportunity to learn about himself. It was clear to me that the source of his frustration was his inability to put up proper boundaries.

After we'd chatted, he had a calm conversation with his mother, explaining it would be helpful if she wrote down a list of everything that needed doing and then, each time he came, he would get them done. To his amazement, his mother thought this was a great idea. Her intention had never been to stress her son out; she simply hadn't considered this alternative.

What helped Brian further was the phrase, 'If you were her, you'd be acting like her.' I asked him to imagine what life must be like for his mother. She was immobile, dependent and a widow whose husband had died a year earlier. She lived by herself and felt scared. The way she was acting wasn't coming from a lack of love for him, but from fear. Once he started to imagine this, his body language visibly changed. His shoulders dropped and he looked pensive and sad.

Over the course of a few months, a daily practice of seeking out friction allowed Brian to take the heightened emotion out of the situation and see it rationally for what it was. He also began to recognize other situations in his life in which he had failed to put up proper boundaries: at work, and with his wife. This transformed Brian. He became much better at speaking up when he was unhappy and at calmly negotiating solutions with the people in his life. His migraines went and he felt less stressed, more in control and more aligned.

How to Deal with Criticism

A common source of social friction is criticism. When we are criticized or feel as if we have been criticized, it can really affect how we feel. If we don't take time to process that emotion and reframe the situation, it can have a negative impact on our work, our focus and our relationships.

The next time you are in this situation, try the following strategies:

- Ask yourself how you are feeling about the criticism. What emotions is it bringing up? For example, do you feel upset, resentful, frustrated or angry? How you feel is how you feel. The important thing is to be honest with yourself and really take time to acknowledge how you are feeling.

- If you have space and time, it may be worth taking a few deep breaths where your exhale is longer than your inhale, in order to calm your nervous system down which will allow you to assess the situation more effectively. For example, you could breathe in for a count of two and breathe out for a count of four – or another breathing cadence that suits you better.

- Now ask yourself why this criticism is bothering you so much? Be as honest as you can.

- Try to feel where this emotion is stored in your body. Many people feel anxiety in their stomach, or stress in their back and neck. If you can identify where the emotion is located, spend a few minutes focusing on your breath. Try to breathe into the part of your body where you feel the emotion and see if you can help the emotion dissipate or ease up. Don't worry if you are unable to do this initially. It gets easier with practice.

- Some people find it useful to think about a 'criticism tea strainer'. The idea is that you visualize straining the comment as if you were straining tea leaves. You leave the emotional reactivity (the tea leaves) behind and allow the comment (the actual tea) to flow through. This allows you to calmly examine the criticism, without the associated negative emotions.

- Now, calmly contemplate what was said. Is there any truth to this critique?

- If there is some truth to it, remember you've been given an opportunity to learn something. What can you do, practically, to prevent such criticism in the future?

- If, after honest evaluation, you don't feel there's any truth to it, try to look at the situation from the other side. Why did that person choose to criticize you unfairly? Were they stressed out in their own lives? Were they jealous of your success because they're insecure about who they are? Do they feel your success threatens their own? Really try to understand what could be behind it. Of course, you may not know for sure, but simply trying to understand can take the sting out of the situation and increase your sense of control. As you know, this sense of control immediately strengthens your Core Happiness.

- Try to find some compassion for your critic. Remember, if you were them, with their upbringing and their life experiences, you'd probably be acting the same way. Also, reflect on the emotion that this is bringing up in you and realize that how you feel is down to you. Nobody else can actually make you feel a thing. You are in control.

- To comfort yourself further, imagine what you might say to a close friend or child if they were being criticized like this.

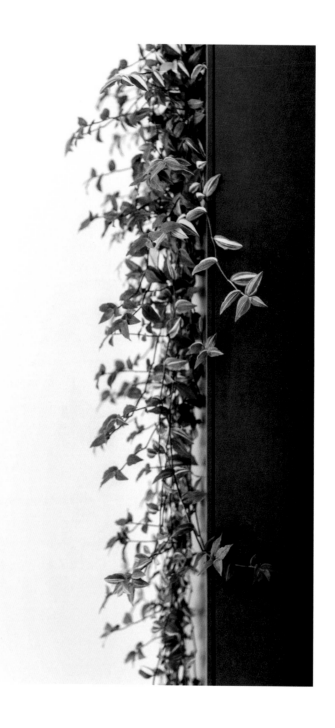

CONCLUSION

Seek out friction wherever you can. See the problems you encounter with the people in your daily life as precious gifts. Hold an honest mirror up to yourself. Use what you see in it to write a new story for yourself, one in which you're a hero, not a victim – a story that empowers you to take control of your own wellbeing. Write a new story for other people, too; one full of empathy and compassion in which everyone is doing the best they can. Remember, you always have a choice in how you react to life's inevitable difficulties. You have a choice in the stories you tell. Why not choose happiness?

№ 6

TALK TO STRANGERS

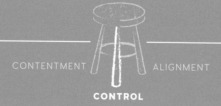

CONTENTMENT   ALIGNMENT

CONTROL

I was born in the north-west of England. Growing up, I'd heard the rumour that people 'down south' weren't very friendly, but I had always dismissed this as a lazy, unfair stereotype. My first opportunity to spend any proper time in the south was when I went to London in my early twenties. I remember getting off the train at Euston station and making my way to the Underground, feeling so excited. The moment I sat down on the Tube train, I began chatting to the person next to me. 'Busy day?' I asked. She gave me a tight-lipped smile and immediately went back to her newspaper. Perhaps, I thought, she was having a bad morning. I made eye contact with the chap on the other side of me and nodded him a quick greeting. He was in his sixties and had a smart black leather briefcase clutched between his knees. For a moment, I actually thought he might reach over and slap me.

It was truly shocking. I'd travelled two hours from my hometown and felt like I'd arrived on another planet. But almost as amazing was how quickly I found myself allowing those initial interactions to change my natural behaviour. As I started coming to the city more regularly, I'd get on the Tube, put my headphones on and create this cone of personal space around me. But this behaviour came at a cost. I soon realized how out of alignment I was being when I acted like this. I'm a natural extrovert. I thrive on social contact. These days, when I'm on the Tube, I will often say hi to a person near me. If I've chosen well, they respond with a smile and a comment. It is amazing how good this feels. It's a shot of pure happiness in the arm, and it's very clear that myself and my new Tube-mate both feel it.

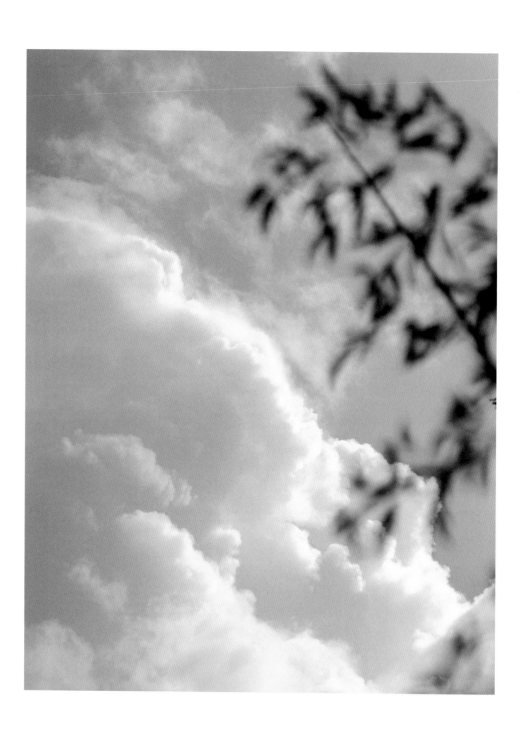

INCREDIBLE VITAMIN S

Why does this moment of micro-connection feel so good? Because humans are social animals. Nature wants us to connect with others and rewards us with positive feelings when we do. Psychologists have found we have a network in our brains that acts as a 'sociometer'. The job of the sociometer is to constantly scan our social world. If it detects we're not securely connected, our self-esteem plummets and our stress response is triggered. We become anxious and unhappy and at greater risk of becoming physically and mentally ill. It's hard to overstate the importance of having a network of positive social connections. One study at Harvard University that's been tracking people for an incredible seventy-five years found that the number-one predictor of happiness and wellbeing over the course of our lives is the quality of our relationships. Nothing else came close.

But relationships come in many different forms. Clearly, it's good to have healthy ties to our romantic partners, family and friends. If we want to keep the Core Happiness stool strong and upright, it's pretty obvious that we ought to also seek positive relations with our bosses and colleagues. If, at work, we're treated with hostility or suspicion, or if we're overlooked and ignored, it will be much more difficult to feel content and in control. What's less obvious is that we should also seek to feel connected to the strangers that flit in and out of our everyday lives. A 2021 study by psychologists Paul van Lange and Simon Columbus found that positive interactions with strangers 'help us serve basic needs such as feeling connected, appreciated, along perhaps with the realization of personal growth in ourselves'. They advised people 'to initiate brief interactions, even a smile, to strangers' because doing so supplies us with a critically important social nutrient they call Vitamin S.

Research by the US psychologist Professor Nicholas Epley backs this up. What I found especially fascinating about Epley's work, given my own experiences, is that it involved studying the behaviour of strangers on trains. He asked commuters in Chicago to do one of three things. The first group was told to keep themselves to themselves, the second group was asked to just do what they would ordinarily, and the third group was asked to do something shocking and radical: to reach out, say 'hello' to someone and have a conversation. Before the test began, he asked his participants how they'd feel if they were made to do the third option. They said they wouldn't like it. Being made to talk to strangers, they thought, would make them enjoy their commute less. They were also asked how many strangers they thought would be receptive to their overtures. They predicted about 40 per cent of commuters would be happy to chat.

So what were the results? Every single one of the strangers they reached out to was glad to connect. And did this connection ruin their journey, as they'd expected? Of course not. Not only were they happier if they made the effort to connect during their journey, that happiness lasted, carrying over into the rest of their day. These simple, regular hits of Vitamin S are powerful because they offer our subconscious minds a continual sense of reassurance. I call it Positive Social Feedback.

Of course, these results did not seem to reflect my initial experiences on the London Underground, but I think there is a simple explanation. London daytime travellers are often highly stressed, rushing from one appointment to the next. For many, that precious time on the Tube with their headphones in may be the only bit of me-time they'll get for hours. I am not suggesting for a minute that we should be intrusive and harass people who don't want to be disturbed. A key part of happiness for ourselves and others is to be respectful to the world around us. It's completely reasonable that many of them don't want to be disturbed.

But how many of them are simply copying what everyone around them is doing? How many are truly happy being zoned off from the world around them? I suspect it's surprisingly few. They're simply responding to the environment around them, assuming the person next to them doesn't want to connect. Humans are social animals and we are wired for connection. Epley has replicated his findings all over the place – in buses, in taxis and in waiting rooms. He's even replicated these findings on commuter trains into London.

My initial negative social encounters on the Tube are now a thing of the past. I quickly realized that it all comes down to being sensitive to social cues. It's easy to see from someone's body language if they're up for a chat. I quickly found that Londoners are no different to the rest of the human race. They're social animals too. These days I strike up conversations almost every time I go down there. And on the rare occasions I misread the signals and get rebuffed, I think of a way to make that person a hero.

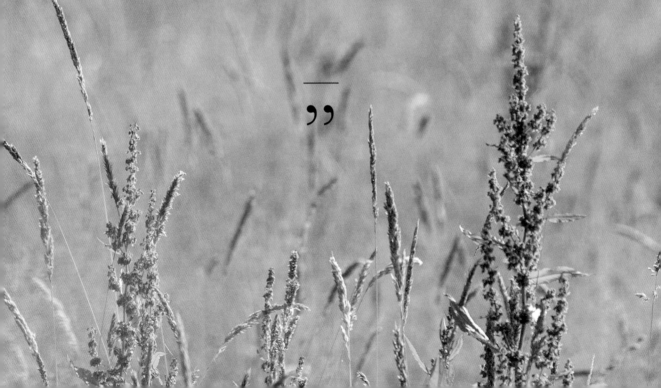

"

Humans are
social animals and
we are wired for
connection.

"

THE COST OF CONVENIENCE

One of the most extraordinary things about Epley's study is what it reveals about the mindset of these typical commuters. They not only expected that most people wouldn't want to connect with them, they predicted they'd be less happy if they did! What has gone wrong with these social animals that they feel so negative about the simple act of being social? I'm convinced a big part of the answer lies in our Want Brain world. Since the end of the Second World War, so many of our efforts have gone into making life more convenient. Advances from the spread of private transport in the middle of the last century to the modern craze for home-delivery shopping have served to make our lives much easier – but a lot less social.

Of course, I'm not advocating a ban on the car or on Amazon or online grocery delivery services. But I am saying there's a huge cost to all this convenience. Whereas once we'd have walked to the local market, passing neighbours multiple times a day, we're now more likely to drive to a large anonymous supermarket or order our groceries on an app. We don't go to the cinema as much; instead, we watch Netflix at home. We don't even queue in person any more. Rather than standing in a line with other humans and having a chat to pass the time, we do our queuing on the phone, listening to a recorded voice telling us how important our call is. Our lives are so busy the commute is often the only time we get to spend 'alone', reading the papers, doing a crossword, getting lost in a book. We're chronically deprived of Positive Social Feedback.

When I was a child and I answered the home landline phone, my mum would make sure that I had a short, polite conversation with whoever was calling before I handed it over. This would never happen now, because everyone has their own personal phone. Technology is slowly but surely erasing unplanned human interaction from everyday life. It's become normal to live with very little social contact. Studies find that people today are twice as lonely as they were in the

1980s and this is having a devastating effect on our physical and mental wellbeing. People who feel lonely are more likely to get a host of chronic illnesses, such as heart disease, depression and anxiety.

This is why I think it's more essential than ever to intentionally seek moments of Positive Social Feedback. We can do this pretty much anywhere. One set of researchers studied people striking up brief conversations with cashiers in Starbucks. They found people who have these chats leave happier and with 'a better sense of belonging with their community' than those who don't. Even brief eye contact with a total stranger has been found to increase feelings of inclusion and belonging.

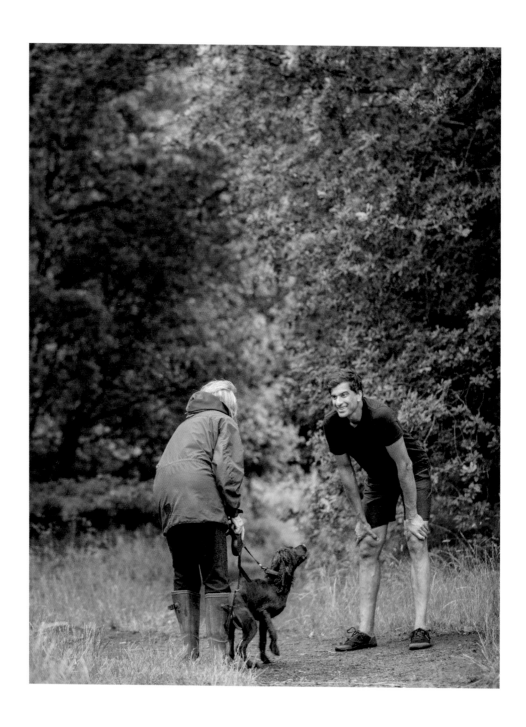

SOCIAL MEDIA IS
SOCIAL THEATRE

If you're thinking you're smashing this rule already because you spend three hours a day communicating with strangers on Instagram and Facebook, I'm afraid I have bad news: social media doesn't count. The problem with online connection is that it mostly takes the form of validation-seeking or conflict. This is baked into the design of these platforms. Strangers tend to connect online because they want something from you – a follow back, an approving comment or, in the worst situations, they're showing off to their followers by attacking you in some way. Online life is transactional. It's connection with benefits. All too often, it's Negative Social Feedback.

Social media also seems to have a terrible, warping effect on social behaviour. There have been so many times I've met people in real life who I knew previously only via social media and found them to be nothing like what I imagined. And it's always the same story – they're nicer. They don't resemble the confrontational, arrogant, hate-inducing persona I've got to know on Twitter. I have come to think of social media as social theatre. People aren't really looking for connection, they're performing in order to get validation. They want love, so they create a persona that gets them more love in that particular environment. They're not behaving in their daily lives as they do online. If they were, they wouldn't get very far. If you start to see social media as social theatre, too, you'll understand it better – and learn to take it a lot less seriously.

CASE STUDY

Thirty-five-year-old Femi came in to see me with a skin condition. He had previously tried various medications with other doctors with limited success. I got the strong sense that there was a lot of background stress in his life and decided to take a different approach.

Femi always seemed very down and dressed scruffily, with stains on his clothes, and struggled to make eye contact. He told me he didn't go out much, and preferred to keep to himself. I asked him if there were any groups or clubs he could join. He admitted he felt awkward and self-conscious around others so would rather stay home. He was happiest when he was in his sunny kitchen in the morning, catching up on the news on his smartphone, drinking coffee.

I gave Femi an unusual prescription: to read a real newspaper each morning instead. He would need to leave the house to go and buy it, and ended up at the local newsagent's. Each morning, he would pop in to pick up the newspaper and be served by the same shop assistant. Little by little, they got to know each other. They would say hi, exchange happy looks and, within days, they formed part of the rhythm of each other's daily lives.

One day, after a couple of weeks, the usual assistant wasn't there as he was suffering with flu. Femi asked after him, and over the following days this small conversation led to bigger conversations which, in turn, led to him getting to know some of the other regulars. Femi was starting to feel part of his local community.

One morning, he ended up chatting with one of the regulars who always came in wearing gym gear and carrying a sports bag. Femi was intrigued and discovered he went to the gym each morning for a Boxercise class at eight. The man invited Femi to join him the following day and, although Femi felt nervous, he went along and loved it. Before he knew it, he was attending regularly and loved the way it made him feel afterwards and the strong sense of community.

The next time I saw Femi, he was like a different man. He'd lost weight, his clothes were neat and clean and he was visibly glowing with happiness. His skin condition had also gone. I can't know for sure whether this was down to my social prescription, but I strongly suspect it was. And all it took to trigger Femi's transformation was a newspaper and a smile.

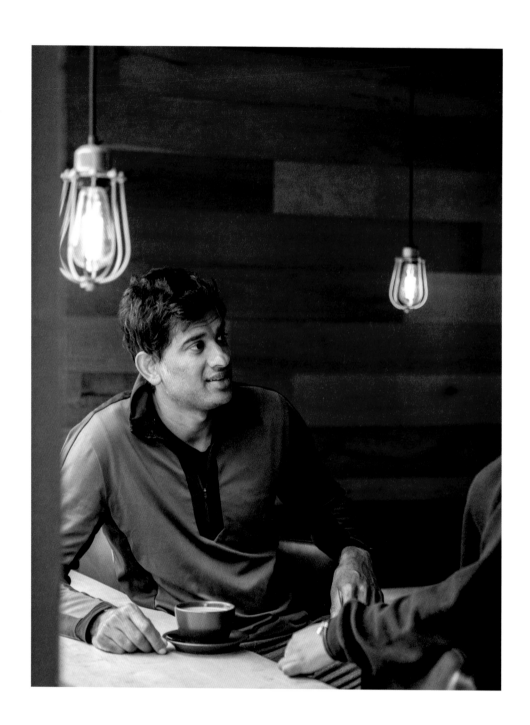

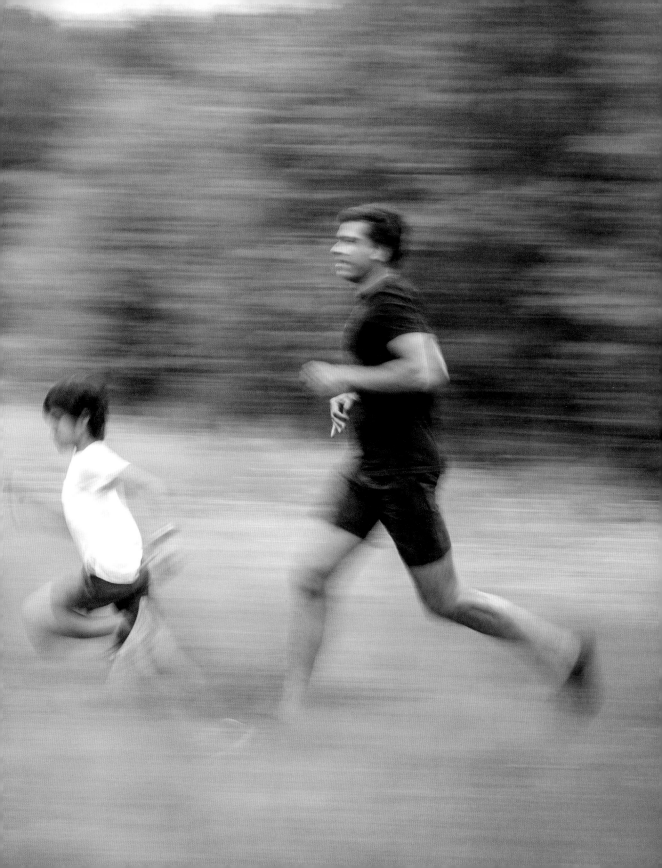

Running with Strangers

I'm a massive fan of parkrun. It started off as a run in south London between friends and has now become a global phenomenon, with more than 2,000 locations in 22 countries across 5 continents. All events are free to enter and delivered by volunteers. I've been going to parkrun with my family for years. Some mornings we don't feel especially motivated, or the weather is really bad, but we know that all we need to do is get to the start line and then, as if by magic, thirty minutes later, we'll have completed a 5k run.

I believe the secret of parkrun's success is that it is not really about running, but community. Just like that other global fitness phenomenon, CrossFit, what keeps people coming back is that sense that they're part of a tribe. They belong. Parkrunners are not necessarily people you'd exchange phone numbers with. They're semi-strangers, living their own lives. But there's something so powerful and life-affirming in seeing the same faces every week – the smiles during the race, the nods of acknowledgement, the unconditional support. Even on a bitterly cold, rainy Saturday in the north of England, going to parkrun lights up our lives. It's a large dose of Positive Social Feedback, and it reminds us that we belong.

Is there a local parkrun where you live? Have you signed up yet? What is stopping you? If parkrun doesn't take your fancy, is there any other group activity you can sign up for that will force you to interact with more 'strangers'. It could be doing the shopping in person at the supermarket rather than online, buying the newspaper at the local newsagent's or having a regular coffee in a café. It could be a weekly in-person yoga or Pilates class in addition to practising by yourself at home. We are social animals. We need to act like them as well.

CONCLUSION

The trick with talking to strangers is to start small. Especially if you're insular and introverted, you can begin with a smile and a moment of eye contact and ratchet up from there. Even the briefest of social contacts counts as Positive Social Feedback. It will make you feel good, more confident and empowered to go for more. No matter how often you talk to strangers right now, I'd like you to start doing it more. Push yourself out of your comfort zone just a little bit. You'll strengthen your Core Happiness by making yourself feel more in control, more content and more aligned. The father of one of my friends is in his eighties and still thriving. He once told me the secret to a long and happy life is to talk to at least ten different people every day. I think he's right.

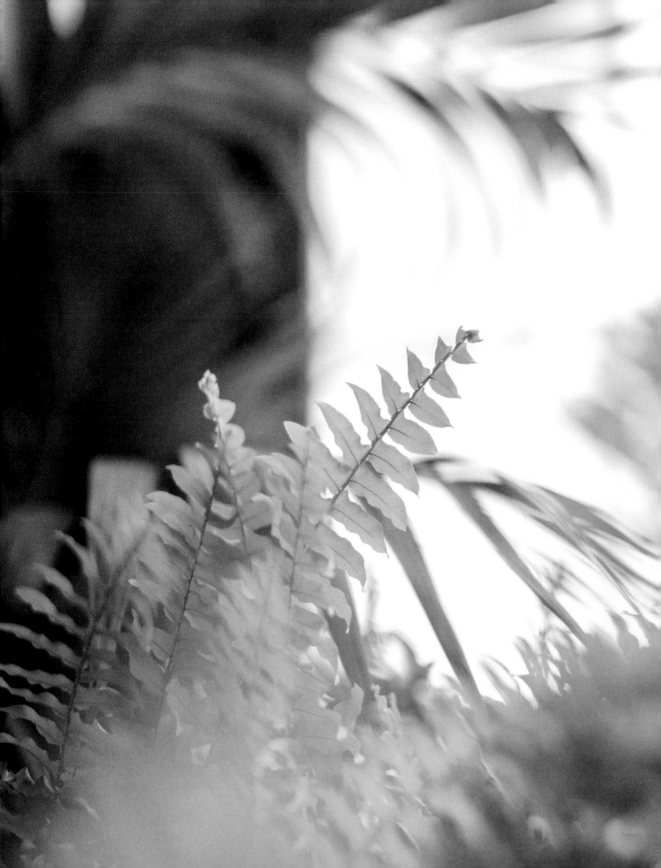

N<u>o</u>. 7

TREAT YOUR PHONE LIKE A PERSON

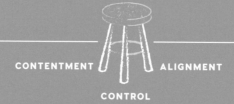

CONTENTMENT ALIGNMENT

CONTROL

Billions of people around the world have a smartphone as a constant companion. It goes pretty much everywhere we do: to work, to the shops, on walks, on holiday, to bed. We take it to dinner – and lunch, and breakfast. We take it to the sofa to watch television with us. Many of us even take it to the bathroom. Modern phones have many incredible benefits, but have we been seduced by all the pros and ignored the many cons? What is the price we have actually paid? For many of us, they have cost us our happiness.

It's no exaggeration to say that our phones have become our electronic shadows. But imagine if your actual shadow made you feel the way your phone does. I find this such a fascinating thought experiment, because it really forces us to consider the incredible power this device has, and the many ways it alters the texture of our everyday lives. If your phone was a person, and that person stressed you out and distracted you as much as your phone does, how would you feel about them? If that person were able to fascinate you, entertain you and titillate you to the extent that your phone can, how would your partner feel about them? How would your children feel about them? Would they really want that person hanging around with you, all of the time?

YOUR ELECTRONIC STALKER

Your loved ones simply cannot compete with modern technology. No human being can. Your phone has a unique record of your history and preferences: every song, every film, every purchase, every intellectual, sexual and social connection you've ever made online. It generates a deep personal knowledge of exactly what triggers your Want Brain and uses that knowledge to draw you into its universe of personally curated distractions. When your loved ones are competing with your phone for attention, they're competing with the might and brilliance of Silicon Valley. These technologists have spent billions of dollars working out how to find the weak spots in human psychology and exploit them. And, make no mistake, they're good at their jobs. If you struggle to manage your relationship with your phone, it's not because you're weak. It's not because you have poor self-control. It's because you're fighting an invisible war with the smartest people on earth.

This is a war for your attention. The more you use one app or another, the more the technologists know about you, and the more advertising revenue they generate. And they don't just target the young: anyone can become prey. One of my elderly relatives is pretty much addicted to his phone. He comes to our house for meals and his phone is there with him at the table. As we're chatting and enjoying the food and each other's company, he's scrolling through WhatsApp and Facebook. He tries to get us to look at messages and watch funny videos, probably as a way of making us feel included in his digital bubble. Of course, what we really want isn't to watch a cat play the piano, but his undivided attention. When he's hanging out with the internet, he's not hanging out with us. Sitting at the dinner table is a social event, and so is gathering around the television as a family. It's a shared experience, little different from being around the tribal campfire and being told an incredible story. As soon as somebody takes their phone out, they've broken the magic circle. They've gone somewhere else.

"

Your loved ones simply cannot compete with modern technology. No human being can.

"

It's only too easy to lose track of the time the technologists steal from us. Earlier, I introduced you to researcher Professor Ashley Whillans of Harvard Business School. Her concept of Time Confetti refers to 'these little seconds and minutes lost to unproductive multi-tasking'. Our phones are clearly responsible for shredding much of our time into confetti. But even when we're not directly interacting with them, they can have a negative effect. Firstly, this is because when we shift from one task to another, we have to use up significant amounts of brain energy to get back to what we were doing before. We can't instantly switch our brain from one task to another and this means there is less brain power left for the important things in our lives, like work and relationships. If we're constantly flipping our attention to and from our phones, we're not going to be concentrating deeply on anything at all.

Secondly, our phones downgrade much of the rest of our time. Even when we're not actually using them, their simple presence can be a distraction. We all know we're less present with our friends when our phone's around – and with our wife, husband, boyfriend, children or job. Research has shown just how powerful these devices are at distracting us. Adults visiting a science museum with their children who reported using their smartphone regularly during the visit enjoyed the experience less than those who reported low smartphone use. In addition, they described feeling more distracted, they derived less meaning from the experience and had reduced feelings of social connection with their children. What this study tells me is that smartphone use isn't simply a harmless bit of fun. Many of life's most magical experiences are corroded and downgraded by them. How many of your relationships and special life moments are being damaged in this way?

It's essential to our Core Happiness that we feel content and in control, yet merely having a phone with us is often enough to damage this. But phones attack another leg of the Core Happiness stool too. How many of us want to be considered a good parent, partner or colleague? The phone, with its incredible power to distract us and downgrade our time and to nudge us closer to our stress threshold, continually pushes us out of alignment with who we want to be.

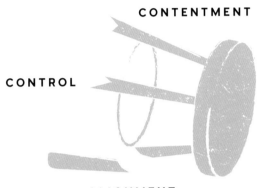

CONTENTMENT

CONTROL

ALIGNMENT

Of course, we've always had temptations to distract us, such as newspapers, TVs and gaming consoles. What makes smartphones different is their portability and power. Most of us are literally never without our devices. Around 80 per cent of adults can reach their phone without moving their feet, twenty-four hours per day. On average, we look at our screens between 200 and 250 times per day. A study by researchers at the University of Texas that involved 800 smartphone users found that their cognitive capacity was 'significantly reduced' when their devices were within reach, even when they were off. As Professor Adam Alter, author of *Irresistible: The Rise of Addictive Technology and the Business of Keeping Us Hooked*, told me on my podcast, if you ask people, 'Would you like things that are on your phone to be implanted into your brain?' most say no. But, because of the fact we're surrounded by them twenty-four hours per day, they're having almost the same effect. According to Adam's research, 40–45 per cent of 20–35-year-olds would rather have a broken bone in their hand than a broken phone.

(To hear my podcast conversation with Professor Adam Alter about the addictive nature of technology, visit www.drchatterjee.com/132.)

"

We smile 30 per cent
less when our phone
is present.

—

"

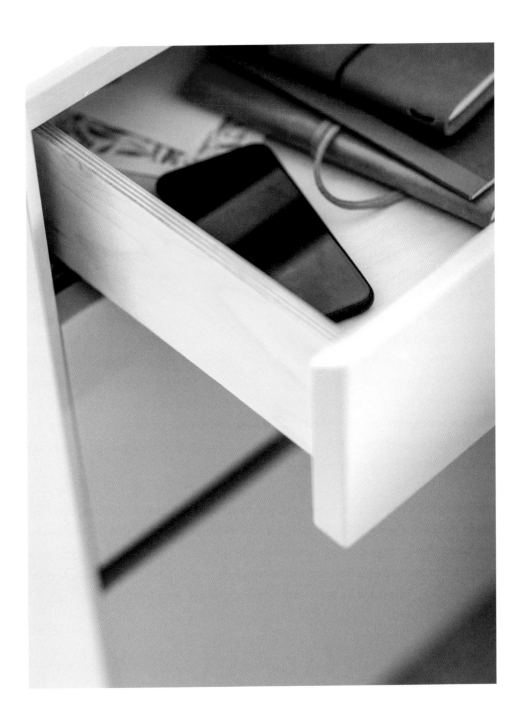

PHONE BRAIN

Don't get me wrong, I'm as vulnerable to the lures of the smartphone as anyone. Social media has become an important part of my job, and there is no question that, at times, I have used it more than I would have liked. A few summers ago, I decided to take three weeks off my social platforms. I deleted the Facebook, Instagram and Twitter apps from my phone. About half an hour after I'd done this, I found myself picking up my phone and ghost-checking them. This continued for the next three days.

One of the most amazing benefits of my social media holiday was that it allowed me to go inside myself and figure out, what do I think about the world? I hadn't realized the extent to which my thoughts were constantly being influenced by online conversations. There's so much groupthink on social media. We sink into these online worlds and don't realize how much our minds are becoming infected with other people's views. Your phone can become like another person that you take with you everywhere you go, whispering thoughts and ideas into your mind. We lose touch with our own thoughts, values and beliefs. If we're not careful, we catch a bad case of Phone Brain, allowing the angriest and most biased pockets of social media to do our thinking for us.

Having regular phone-free time is essential for our wellbeing. Whether that be fixed periods each day or longer periods several times per year, the effects can be profound. You start to quieten down the external noise and hear the signals your own body is sending you. You start to become more in touch with yourself. And, as you do so, this helps you be more in touch and present with those around you.

WHAT WE'VE LOST

It's one of those unfortunate quirks of the human condition that it's very hard to imagine what we've lost. How would your life have been different over the last ten years if you hadn't had your phone? How would your relationship with your partner, kids, boss or friends be different? Would you be more or less angry at the world? Would you feel more content, more in control and more aligned? The psychologist Professor Laurie Santos, of Yale University in Connecticut, finds that 'just deciding to stay off social media will have a bigger effect on your happiness than earning $100,000 or marrying the love of your life'. Other research has found we smile 30 per cent less when our phone is present. I find these facts truly upsetting. When I contemplate all the precious moments I've lost over the years, it can honestly bring me close to tears.

 (To listen to my podcast conversation with Professor Laurie Santos, visit www.drchatterjee.com/151.)

CASE STUDY

Lydia, forty-one, was struggling with her marriage, and she came to see me because this was making her feel low and depressed. She would often come home and spend hours on her phone answering work emails. She'd also stay up late binge-watching videos on YouTube or endlessly scrolling through Instagram as she couldn't face going to bed, then waking up to the same tedium the following day. Her husband was becoming frustrated that every time he wanted to interact with her she would be distracted and looking at her devices. He felt ignored, unloved and unheard. This emotional tension underpinned all of their interactions and often led to seemingly unrelated arguments.

After talking to Lydia, it was clear to me that she was using her work as a distraction. Things were not going well in her relationship and, instead of tackling them, it was easier to use the excuse of work. There is also something about the ubiquitous nature of phones. In my experience, doing work emails while sitting down at a desk with a laptop does not appear to have as negative an effect on our relationships as half-looking on our phones while also trying to interact with our partner.

I explained to Lydia that having her phone around while trying to interact with her husband was like having a third person in the room. Lydia, like so many of us, found it hard to resist looking at her phone. I suggested that she take the work email app off her phone, as well as her social media apps, to reduce temptation. I also recommended that she go on a long walk every weekend with her husband without their phones.

It's no exaggeration to say this transformed their relationship and their lives. It took time, for sure. But, little by little, they started connecting again. Because Lydia and her husband had created time to be present with one another, they were able to air any niggles. They had space to listen to each other without the option of running away to Instagram or email. Within weeks, their relationship improved. They were happier, and more intimate. Neither Lydia nor her husband had realized the destructive impact their phones were having on their relationship.

REPLACE STEPS

One of the cardinal rules of creating new habits is to make any behaviour you want to introduce into your life as easy as possible to do. If you make something easy to do, you are much more likely to do it. This is exactly how the technologists get us addicted to their products. Our phones and apps become compulsive because they create a strong desire for Junk Happiness, whether it's to alleviate boredom, for social validation or for something to buy, and then make it as easy as possible to satisfy the Want Brain's urge. Amazon's 'one click' ordering system is a classic example of this. It has had a huge impact on their profits because it makes getting Junk Happiness incredibly easy.

The best way to fight back against the technologists is by putting steps back in. If an app is causing you problems, then delete that app. At the very least, turn off the notifications so you use it only when you need to, and not when it wants you to. Make it harder for yourself to use that product or service. For me, deleting the email app from my phone was a game-changer, and one of the most impactful things I've done for my wellbeing over the past few years. It made me realize that I really don't need email on my phone. It's almost never the case that an email arrives that has to be dealt with absolutely immediately – if there's an emergency, someone will phone. Emails have the potential to disturb my walks when I want to be enjoying nature, my train journeys when I want to be reading, and my time with the kids when I'm with them in the park. I now only look at emails when I'm sitting down at my laptop, when I intentionally decide I want to.

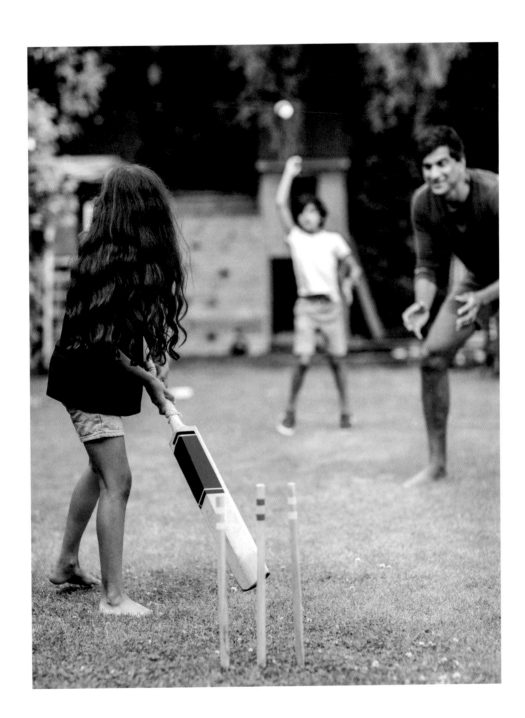

5 Ways to Create Distance from Your Phone

Here are some ways you can put steps back in that make it less likely that your phone will interfere with the important things in your life:

1. **Look at what apps are on your phone and ask yourself which ones bring you value and which ones don't.** Consider removing those you don't really need. Consider all of them, including email. Don't assume you can't live without these apps. Experiment and see what happens. For example, if you want to spend less time on social media, delete all of your social media apps from your smartphone. You can still access them when you want from your laptop or even the browser on your phone, but not having the app on your phone makes it just a little bit harder to access. I did this a while back with Twitter and Facebook and now find myself hardly ever on those platforms. And do I miss them? Not one bit!

2. **Customize your home screen.** If deleting the apps feels like a step too far, consider putting the ones that you want to use less in a folder on your phone and move that folder away from your home screen. This makes it much less likely you will get distracted and find yourself mindlessly using them. One of my friends did this with WhatsApp, Messenger and Instagram and now uses them only when he really wants to. He says that this one move alone has had a dramatic effect on his own wellbeing and on his relationship with his wife.

3. **Turn off all notifications from apps like social media and email.**
    Notifications result in you being at the beck and call of the technologists,
    who want your attention on their platforms to sell you things and advertise
    to you. The people you value who really need to speak to you will likely
    message or call you directly, so removing the constant pings from multiple
    apps puts you back in control. This is one of the simplest, yet most effective
    things you can do. I did this over five years ago and, along with deleting the
    work email app on my phone, it is the most impactful thing I have done to
    improve my relationship with technology. (Of course, if you have an app that
    you feel is helpful for you and your wellbeing – for example, a meditation
    app – consider keeping notifications on to help remind you to engage in the
    behaviour.)

4. **Put your phone in a different room when doing intense work that needs
    your full concentration.** This is deceptively effective. Often, we will
    reflexively look at our phones because they are next to us. As soon as we get
    bored or a little frustrated with our work, it is all too easy to pick up the
    phone and distract ourselves. Just having to get up and move rooms is often
    all it takes to reduce our usage. When I am in deep flow when writing books
    like this one, I make sure my phone is nowhere near me and, since doing so,
    my productivity has improved immeasurably.

5. **Get friendly with the Do Not Disturb function.** Learn to use your phone's
    Do Not Disturb settings. Each phone is unique but most of them will allow
    you to program them so you can stop all notifications, calls and texts from
    reaching you when you don't want to be disturbed. For example, this could be
    while you are driving, working or during mealtimes.

IS YOUR SMARTPHONE MAKING YOU HAPPIER?

A smartphone is built for being on the move. That's why, in the UK at least, we call it a 'mobile'. If this seems like a ridiculously obvious thing to point out, let me ask you – why do you have it switched on at home? Many of us still have a landline for phone calls, although this is rapidly declining. You probably have a computer or laptop somewhere through which you can access the internet. You may also have a radio or even a CD player to listen to music. At home, the tools to do those jobs have their place, and they stay in their place. You're forced to engage with them intentionally. This means you're more likely to use them when you really want to and need to, rather than simply to fill your time when you get a little bit bored. I want you to be more intentional with your use of your phone and start thinking about it as if it was another person. Do you always want that person walking around with you, everywhere you go?

Have you ever thought about turning your mobile phone off when you're at home? If this sounds too tough, perhaps you could try it just in the evenings at first, then work up from there. This is a strategy I often use myself. I still keep a landline at home, and only my family and close friends have access to the number. This means it's really easy for me to disengage with my phone when I'm at home. I can turn it off and leave all its noise and temptations behind, which means I can be much more present with my wife and children. If one of my family or friends really needs me, they will always be able to get me on my landline.

I appreciate that everyone has different personal and professional requirements from their phone and that there is no one-size-fits-all. But for many of us, we have simply bought the latest smartphone and allowed it to infiltrate every aspect of our lives without actually thinking about what we really need from it. Most of them, these days, come loaded with many of the latest apps, which are designed to steal your attention. So why not take some time to ask yourself what do you really need from your phone? What things do you do on your phone that really enhance your life rather than take away from it?

Phones can be incredible devices that provide us with a host of different benefits – as long as we are in control of them, rather than them being in control of us. Most of us need our phones for calls and texts. Some of us like the access to music and podcasts as well. But what about everything else? Do you really need all of the apps that you currently have on your phone? Perhaps you could get away with just a maps app to help you get around when out and about and WhatsApp so you can stay in touch with your friends? I understand that there are many occasions when having a variety of different apps on your phone appears to be helpful, but when thinking about technology, we like to overly emphasize the positives and wilfully ignore the negatives. Remember, your smartphone is probably having a negative impact on some of your most important relationships.

There is a growing number of people who, having realized the negative impact that smartphones are having on their lives, are turning their backs on them. They are reverting back to simpler phones that do calls and texts only. Some of these phones are being designed with a few life-enhancing extras, like music and a camera, but without any access to the internet. Being constantly connected to the web everywhere you go makes it incredibly difficult to switch off and be present.

I personally know people who have reverted to these simpler phones, and they tell me they would never go back to a smartphone. They feel calmer, less stressed and less anxious. They also feel more present within their lives and find that the quality of their close relationships has improved. One of my close friends has gone back to an old-fashioned flip-phone which only has calls and texts. He does have a smartphone but keeps it in a drawer at home without a SIM card in it. Whenever he needs to travel long distances and feels he would benefit from the smartphone's functionality, he takes out the SIM card from his flip-phone and pops it into his smartphone for his travels. He has found what works for him because he has taken the time to think about it.

You may find the idea of going without a smartphone too much, and I genuinely don't think everyone needs to. You and your life are unique. But when did you last ask yourself what you really want and need your phone for? Are smartphones really as great as they seem, or are they taking more away from us than they give?

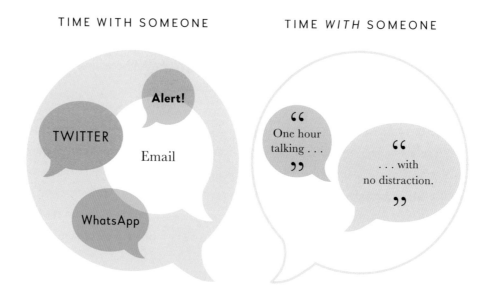

TIME WITH SOMEONE

Alert!

TWITTER

Email

WhatsApp

TIME *WITH* SOMEONE

"One hour talking . . ."

". . . with no distraction."

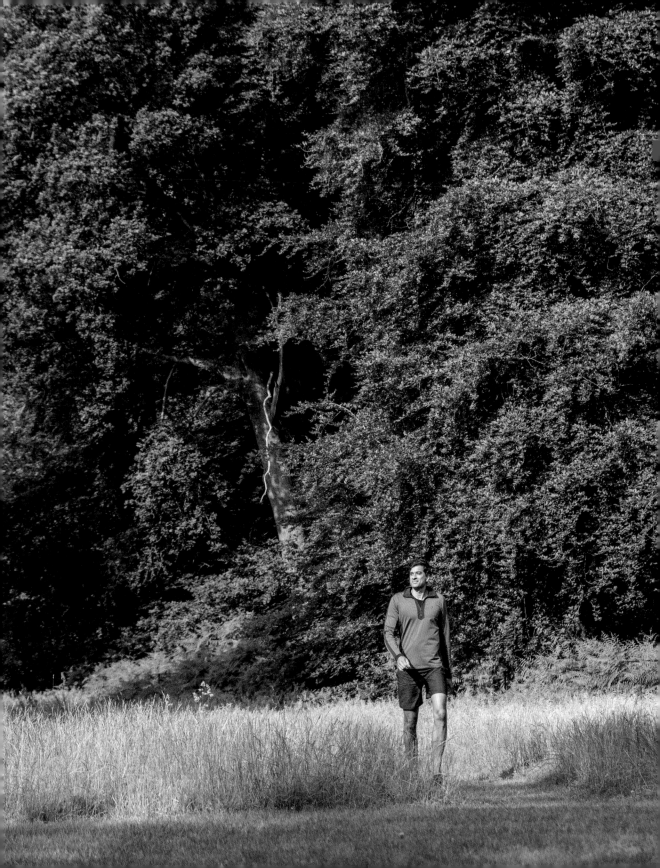

Write Your Phone Norms

All humans have rules for how to live that have evolved slowly over the centuries. Psychologists call these 'norms'. We have norms that we don't spit in the street, for example, or turn up to a social engagement drunk or with an uninvited guest, or eat more than our fair share of food at a buffet. Sitcoms like *Seinfeld* and *Curb Your Enthusiasm* derive much of their comedy from putting a spotlight on these norms and questioning them. But norms are crucial. They tell us how to live with other humans in a place of mutual understanding and respect.

Because smartphones are so new, we haven't yet had the chance to develop norms around them. It's not seen as especially bad when someone pulls out their device during a social occasion. But you'd never whip out a television at a family meal, put it on the table and start watching it. So why would you whip out your phone?

I'd like you to write out five phone norms, for you and your household – perhaps you could decide on them together.

Here are some examples to get you started:

- When out and about with others, put your phone in a bag so it's just a little bit harder to access than it is in your pocket.

- Designate phone-free times in your house (e.g., mealtimes, one hour before bed and one hour first thing in the morning).

- Designate phone-free areas (e.g., the bedroom, the living room or the toilet).

- If you feel you need your phone in your bedroom, perhaps put it in a drawer on the other side of your room so it's a little bit harder to mindlessly grab it.

- Think about times you can go out with your partner, friends or family without your phone. This could be for walks in nature or even a trip to the shops.

- Consider having a work phone and a personal phone. Because our work and personal lives happen via the same devices, it can be challenging to put boundaries in place. Having separate devices can be a solution.

- Consider not using your phone in front of your children. I am very particular about this and will pretty much always go to a different room when I'm contacted or use it when they're not around, as I don't want to give them the signal that my phone is more important than them.

- When you go out for dinner, consider making it a rule that the first person to look at their phone pays the bill.

- If you like using certain apps for music, podcasts, meditation, etc., while at home, consider putting the phone on airplane mode while using them.

The Hidden Porn Epidemic

Pornography is a subject that makes many people feel deeply uncomfortable. But our discomfort in discussing it hides the fact that it has become a major problem. Pornography websites are some of the most popular websites on the planet, with two of them featuring in the top ten of most-visited global websites. Just as concerning, a Swedish study found that 65 per cent of high-school girls aged sixteen had at least some experience of consuming pornography. For high-school boys, the equivalent figure was 96 per cent, with 70 per cent watching once per week and 10 per cent every day.

The internet has given us access to all the titillation we could possibly imagine, and more. Every sexual curiosity or desire can be satisfied in seconds. This attacks two legs of the Core Happiness stool. Firstly, it can make us discontented with our relationships. The simple reality is that pornography is changing our perception of what's normal when it comes to sex and giving us unrealistic expectations of our partners. And it results in many people feeling inadequate and incapable, as they find it impossible to physically compete with what they see online. Without wanting to, we become less content with our partners and less content with ourselves. Porn use also pushes us out of alignment – very few people feel good about themselves afterwards.

CASE STUDY

I've seen from my work as a GP that internet porn is having a huge negative impact on people's wellbeing. I've seen it end long-term relationships and marriages and I've come across many people who've become addicted to it. One of my patients is a 20-year-old man called Max who felt so bad about his habit he couldn't look at me while telling me about it. He accessed pornography websites two to three times a day and felt deeply ashamed.

I spent time with Max, trying to understand what was going on in his life. I soon realized that his porn use was a classic example of Junk Happiness. Max was lacking deep connection with others, had no hobbies or passions and felt lonely. This was affecting how he felt about himself so, understandably, online pornography made him feel good – in the moment. But he'd always feel bad afterwards. This was leading to a negative spiral in which he'd binge on sugar, drink more alcohol and slump on his sofa for hours.

He'd tried mustering the willpower to stop, but he would last only one week at most. Discipline wasn't Max's problem. His porn addiction was a symptom, not a cause. The actual cause was a lack of connection and passion. In addition, the shame he felt around his habit was proving toxic.

Shame thrives in secrecy and, out of that secrecy, addiction is born. When I told Max that I'd seen many patients just like him, I could see he immediately felt much better.

When discussing various options with him, the only activity that sparked a twinkle in his eye was boxing. There was clearly something about it he felt attracted to, even if he was apprehensive about trying. When he did, he found he loved the camaraderie and no-nonsense approach to discipline. He told me, 'In the past, if someone had asked me to do ten squats, I'd have quit after one or two. But in the boxing gym ten means ten.'

What did boxing give Max? It gave him a tribe, a strong sense of purpose and fully immersive time without his phone. It helped him strengthen all three legs of the Core Happiness stool. He became more content, more in control and, most importantly, more aligned – this was the type of person he wanted to be. Soon, without him even having to try, his porn use fell away. It no longer felt consistent with being the proud and strong young man he was fast becoming.

Tips for Reducing Porn Use

Unhealthy pornography usage is a massive hidden problem. If it's affecting you, here are some tips that may help.

- Tell someone about it: shame thrives in secrecy.

- Don't go to bed with your phone. Charge it in a different room and buy a stand-alone alarm clock if you need one.

- Focus on healthy lifestyle habits such as good nutrition, sleep and regular movement. If you look after yourself, you're less likely to feel tired, hungry and emotionally fragile.

- Engage regularly in a passion that nourishes you emotionally.

- Get an accountability buddy. Find someone you trust and open up to them with full honesty. Arrange regular phone calls for support.

- Have a go-to alternative when you feel the urge to consume. This could be phoning a friend, going out for a walk or finding your kids and giving them a cuddle.

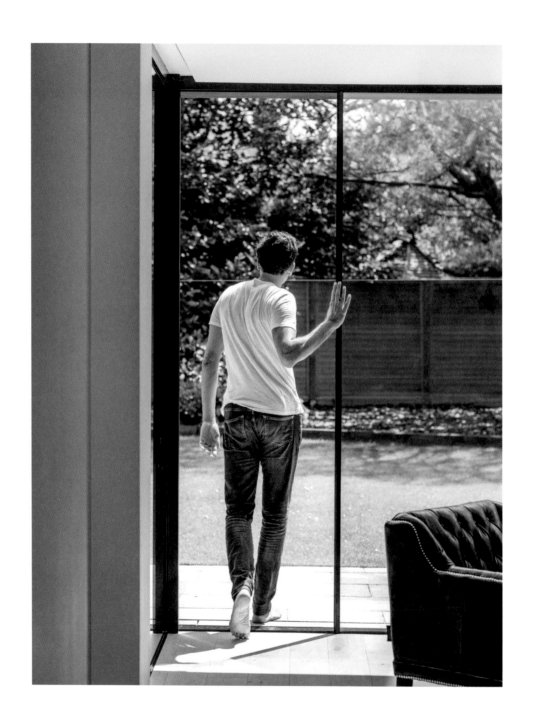

CONCLUSION

Treating your phone like a person will transform your relationship with portable technology. This is a consciousness-raising exercise that'll help you identify the many ways your device silently damages your relationships and weakens your Core Happiness. Setting firm boundaries around the ways your digital shadow is allowed to interfere with you, your life and your loved ones is an essential step to making you feel more content, more in control, and much more aligned. The time has come to power-off for happiness.

HAVE
MASKLESS
CONVERSATIONS

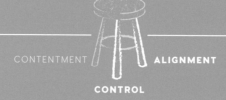

CONTENTMENT   ALIGNMENT

CONTROL

When I was in my twenties, I believed a doctor should be a certain way. They should wear a long white coat, have a stethoscope draped around their neck and speak in an authoritative tone using learned medical jargon. I'm exaggerating, of course, but only a little. It didn't take me long to realize that I'd got this completely wrong. Instead of making me appear trustworthy and impressive, this 'doctor act' I was putting on would often come across as forbidding and distant. As soon as I dropped it and began showing more of who I really was as a person I found myself able to create a truly intimate bond with my patients. They'd sit forward and listen during consultations, and so would I. This would lead to more enjoyable interactions for both myself and my patients. It led to better health outcomes as well.

When I began hosting my weekly podcast just over four years ago, I made the same discovery all over again. I started off with a lot of preconceptions about how a podcast host should be, especially a medical one. But I quickly found that the more I relaxed and revealed myself, including the parts of me I was fearful about putting on public display, the more powerful and rejuvenated I felt. Not only did I get more from each conversation, my listeners did as well. These days the conversations I have on my weekly show are like a lot of my GP consultations – raw, honest, intimate and deeply meaningful. They are, in a word, maskless.

A TIME FOR MASKS AND
A TIME FOR RISKS

There is a place for social masks. Sometimes disguising who we really are and how we're really feeling is exactly the right decision. Earlier, we explored the power of talking to strangers, and discovered how daily doses of Positive Social Feedback can help nudge the brain into thinking it's in a safe environment. If we're not in the mood for socializing when we are out interacting with the world, most of us will choose to wear a disguise of happiness and respect. But we should make sure that we don't end up wearing our masks too often. The French author François de La Rochefoucauld wrote, 'We're so accustomed to disguising ourselves to others that in the end we become disguised to ourselves.' I couldn't agree more.

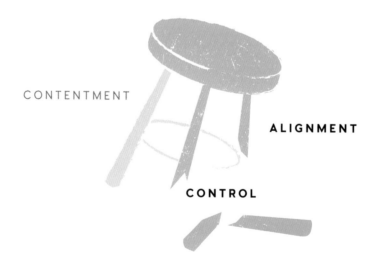

It's all too easy to spend so long in our masks that we forget who we are. When this happens, we knock out two legs of the Core Happiness stool. It becomes impossible for us to live in alignment and we feel out of control because the world feels like an unsafe place, as we are unable to show up as our true selves. We feel that we have to hide who we really are in order to be accepted by others. This is why I believe regular maskless conversations are a must. Not only do maskless conversations allow us to reveal ourselves to others, we learn to understand ourselves better as well.

It's usually with our closest friends and family that we're most easily able to take off our masks. We can reveal who we are without fear of judgement and criticism. When you have a maskless conversation you're completely exposing yourself without trying to impress, entertain or seek validation. They're risky conversations because you don't know for certain how the person listening is going to respond. They're rarely quick and easy and, sometimes, they can be highly emotional, especially if you're opening up about mistakes, regrets and personal traumas. But you always feel differently after you've had a maskless conversation, as if your load has been lightened.

When we don't engage in regular maskless conversations we start to lose touch with who we really are. We feel isolated and lonely. This can have a devastating effect on our mental wellbeing as well as our physical health. The latest scientific research shows us that loneliness is associated with higher rates of depression, anxiety and suicide and has harmful effects on our physical health that are comparable to smoking. It also significantly increases the risk of us getting sick and dying earlier. Having seen tens of thousands of patients over the past two decades, I firmly believe that having regular maskless conversations is as important for your health as the food that you eat.

"

It's only when we understand who we really are that we open up the possibility of becoming the person we wish to be.

—

"

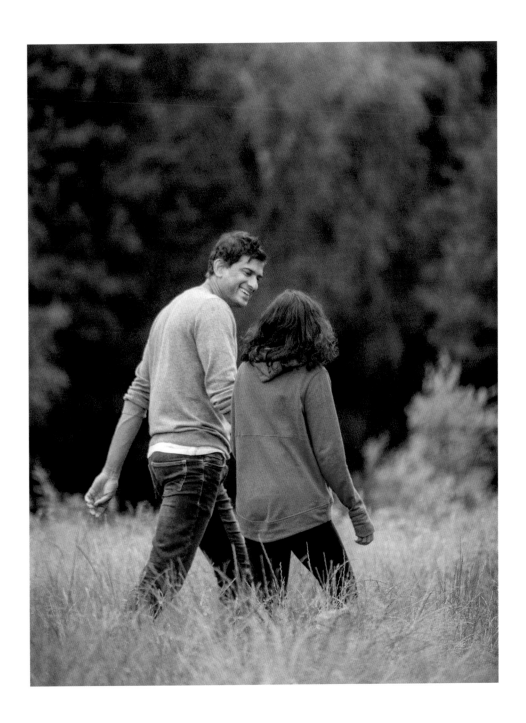

CASE STUDY

From the outside, it looked as if 37-year-old Stuart was crushing life. He was working hard, running his own business and drove a sports car. But, on the inside, he was struggling. He came in to see me because he was feeling low. Sometimes he'd lie in bed in the morning and couldn't face getting out of bed. Sometimes, he'd just slump on his sofa in despair. He felt indifferent to life and lacked motivation. I asked him what things he did to have fun, and he said he didn't. Not only did he not have time for passions, he just didn't get any enjoyment from anything. Late at night, he'd binge on TV until the early morning. This would affect his sleep and he would often wake up feeling exhausted.

Stuart lived in the town where he had grown up and was fortunate that a lot of his schoolmates still lived nearby. He was too busy with work to catch up with them in person but told me he 'saw' them all the time on social media and felt he was up to date with them and their lives. I explained to him that seeing them on social media was not the same thing as seeing them in person, and I suggested that he get together with them face to face, at least once a week.

He came back to see me six weeks later with a huge smile on his face. He was completely transformed. He had started meeting them every Sunday morning in the local café. He'd told them how he was feeling, and they'd had no idea. From what they had been seeing on social media, he was living the perfect life. His honesty triggered honesty in return, and they all began valuing their time together much more. After a few weeks, one of them suggested a weekly game of five-a-side.

Within about three months, the ripple effect had truly kicked in. Stuart's Core Happiness had strengthened dramatically as he felt more content and more in control of his life. Even after the toughest of weeks, he knew he could soon unwind and de-stress with his buddies. He also felt more aligned. He was becoming the person who he really wanted to be. Because of all this, he no longer felt compelled to stay up late watching box sets. His revitalized enthusiasm for five-a-side gave him more motivation to look after his sleep and wider health. After the first few games, he'd been utterly exhausted. This pushed him to start eating better, sleeping better and walking for forty-five minutes every lunchtime to improve his fitness. And it all began with a maskless conversation.

When You Can't Meet, Pick Up the Phone

It's not always going to be possible to have a maskless conversation in person. You might think the second-best option would be a video call. After all, on FaceTime, Zoom or Skype you get to see as well as speak. But I find, as do many of us, that video calls have the surprising effect of reducing intimacy. This is partly because we have the experience of being filmed, which creates a natural anxiety about how we appear. This anxiety is magnified by the fact that we see a live, moving picture of ourselves in the corner of the screen.

Also, we are not actually making real eye contact when on video calls – to do so, you would have to look directly at the webcam at the top of your device, which would mean looking at a camera and not a face. In addition, there's a very slight time delay, which causes us to struggle with social cues. Because of this, we often find ourselves speaking over each other or enduring unnaturally long silences. This can make these calls incredibly tiring as our brains don't receive the social cues they have evolved to receive and so have to work harder to try to find them.

If all that wasn't enough, psychologists have found that we're wired to experience discomfort when we see a face that the brain interprets as being close to ours. According to Jeremy Bailenson, director of Stanford University's Virtual Human Interaction Lab, this often leads to video calls activating the fight-or-flight response. 'From an evolutionary standpoint, if there was a very large human face close by to you, and it was staring right in your eyes, you were likely going to engage in conflict or mating,' he says. This is not a great environment in which to have an intimate conversation.

For many of us, the best way to communicate, when we can't meet in the flesh, is with an old-fashioned phone call. Ideally, it'll be a landline, located in a quiet room where there are few distractions and nobody is likely to interrupt you. When I was young, this was the only way I could talk to my friends when I wasn't actually with them. I've recently rediscovered the joy of the spontaneous phone call. A surprise, unscheduled five-minute catch-up with a mate is enough to give me a major boost of energy and happiness, and a serious, maskless conversation is more nourishing still. Speaking on the landline enables you to dial down your senses and get lost in the call, so all you're consciously aware of are the voices of two people who mean the world to each other.

There is nothing inherently wrong with catching up on a mobile phone. The problem, as we discovered in the last chapter, is that it's extremely easy to fall into the trap of checking your emails or scrolling the web at the same time. Have you ever found yourself doing this? Being even a little bit distracted when having a conversation makes intimacy and taking off masks close to impossible.

(To be clear, I completely understand that video calls have other benefits, like being able to see friends and family who live far away. And, for some people, they can absolutely have intimate conversations through this medium. Just be aware, though, that for many of us they may not be as intimate as we think.)

THE PARADOX OF
AUTHENTICITY

At this point, you might be forgiven for thinking I'm going to start talking up the benefits of being 'authentic'. Surely this is what we're doing when we choose to go maskless? 'Authenticity' is the word of the moment. Many people I know and admire are actively trying to live more authentic lives. But I think this is potentially a much more complex and problematic concept than it first appears. Because it's quite hard to pin down what our 'authentic' self actually is. Is it the person we want to be – the happier and stronger version of us – that we're trying to get to? Or is it the person we truly are right now, with all our flaws and insecurities?

If we decide it's who we are right now, does that mean we're being 'authentic' when we're acting out our flaws? And is this supposed to be a good thing? If so, being 'authentic' seems to give us permission to be rude and thoughtless and to trample over other people's wellbeing. It also gives us permission not to change. For example, is telling the waiter that you thought they were rude and dismissive being authentic? Or is keeping your mouth shut more authentic because you value kindness and treating other people with respect?

So perhaps, instead, our 'authentic' self is the ideal version of us that we're trying to become. But if this is the case, it means being 'authentic' is the same as pretending we're someone we're not. Now, I'm definitely not against 'faking it until you make it', when the circumstances are right. But this isn't what we're trying to achieve when we have a maskless conversation. Maskless conversations are about stepping into your vulnerability. They're about having the courage to be your true self. They're about opening up about your innermost feelings, flaws and insecurities.

Maskless conversations should happen at the right time, with the right people. They usually take place in the presence of people you trust and feel safe with, at least when you start. Otherwise, you can unwittingly fall into an 'authenticity trap', in which you overshare without proper boundaries and start to move away from true authenticity and into performative authenticity.

Some people think that sharing every aspect of themselves, no matter how shocking and raw, is being authentic. They perform authenticity by exaggerating 'realness' to get attention – maximizing their problems and minimizing their privileges. This is about as far from true authenticity as you can get and it can be incredibly dangerous.

When we get lots of positive feedback for doing this, we're incentivized to keep on doing it – stuck in a cycle of wallowing and even celebrating our problems and shortcomings. We reinforce the inner belief that only a fake and manicured version of ourselves is worthy of validation. And if we receive negative comments when we expose our deepest insecurities and flaws, it's going to sting and hurt. We'll feel rejected, and this can make it less likely that we'll open up again. When this happens, we'll respond by putting on even more masks, in the belief that the only way to get on in the world is to be someone we're not. This has a devastating effect on our Core Happiness because we're not living in alignment and our lives feel out of control. And, over time, we feel less content.

INTEGRITY IS THE CURE

Authenticity seems like a worthy aim, but too much of it these days is merely performative. That's why, whenever you think of authenticity, I want you also to think of integrity. Integrity is about being honest with yourself and others. It requires you to practise true authenticity, allowing you to acknowledge and understand who you really are right now while at the same time allowing you to show up in the world as the person who you want to be. When we act with integrity, we know who we currently are, with all of our insecurities, worries and fears – but we're also aware of the person we're trying to become.

The latest research shows that, although we're all unique individuals, we're actually not as different as we might like to think. No matter who we are, when we act in a way that's calm, content, loving, kind, in the present moment and enthusiastic, we feel as if we're being our authentic selves. Expressing every negative thought and acting out every desire as it happens is not when we feel our most authentic.

The truth is that every single one of us is a work in progress. We all have aspects of our personality we'd like to improve. That's completely OK. What's important is that we understand our true self. The only way to truly do this is by acting with integrity. This is exactly what happens in a maskless conversation. We're able to be ourselves. We're being respectful to the person we want to be, but at the same time being honest and vulnerable. We're exposing the parts of ourselves that we sometimes keep locked away deep inside us and being open about our inner struggles and flaws. It's only when we understand who we really are that we open up the possibility of becoming the person we wish to be. As the psychotherapist Carl Rogers said, 'The curious paradox is that when I accept myself just as I am, I can change.'

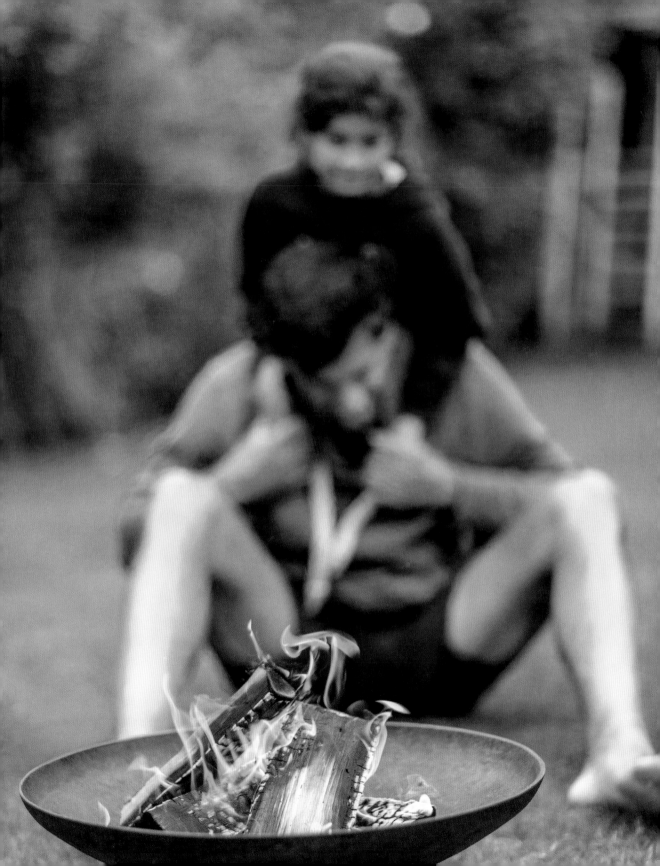

Expand Your Mask-free Zone

Taking off our masks can be frightening. We're often afraid to reveal ourselves for who we really are. We're scared that if other people truly knew us, we'd be rejected. When we become too scared about other people's judgements, the mask we wear becomes permanently glued to us and we begin to fool even ourselves.

If this sounds like you, I'd like to strongly encourage you to start peeling off your social mask more often. Challenge yourself. Think of it this way: there's a cost to not showing others who you really are. What you don't share about yourself, other people will make up in their own minds. They'll create stories about you that are often false and unfair. If you're worried about other people's judgements, remaining hidden can actually be the worst thing you can do.

I'd like you to think about where in your life you can start to take off some of your masks. Here are some examples to get you thinking:

- For many years, it's been considered professionally appropriate to wear a mask at work. But this is slowly starting to change. I think this is a good thing. If a trusted colleague asks how you are, you could choose to say, 'Actually, not great today. My little girl was up with a cough last night and I feel whacked and a little irritable.' If you're coming from a place of integrity, your colleague won't reject you. They'll be more likely to sympathize, empathize and forgive any erratic behaviour later in the day. It's no coincidence that we're seeing a growing trend of companies embracing honesty and that leaders are sharing their insecurities with staff.

- One CEO I know starts every executive Zoom meeting with each team member spending two minutes sharing something that is going on with them outside of work. Everyone on the call is happy to participate. Even though it takes up a quarter of the sixty-minute meeting, they have found that productivity, connection and wellbeing improve dramatically as a result.

- Another simple way to experiment with this is to do a three-word check-in at the start of any work interaction or meeting – simply share three words that describe how you are doing. They do not need to be positive – they are just words that allow people to get a deeper insight into the human they are interacting with for a moment.

5 Questions to Ask Yourself Before Removing Your Mask

Taking off your masks can be done in many different ways, depending on the situation. It could be a really deep, intimate conversation with one of your closest friends, or it could simply be revealing a little bit more about you and your wider life while at work.

No matter where or when you choose to proceed, you may find the following five questions helpful.

1. Is this a safe space to remove my mask?

2. Is this the right medium (in person, on the phone, online, with the kids around, etc.)?

3. Am I exaggerating in any way to gain more attention?

4. Why am I sharing this information right now?

5. Have all parties blocked off enough time for me to truly open up and give this matter the attention and time it deserves?

MASKLESS MEDICINE

As we have already learned, taking off our masks is powerful medicine for our health and happiness. But so is providing space for others to take off theirs. In my first week as a GP, a 20-year-old woman called Kelly came to see me as she was feeling low and indifferent about life. She struggled with her motivation and was worried she 'had depression'. I was very junior as a GP at the time. My guidelines pointed me towards prescribing her an antidepressant. But this didn't feel right. I wanted to understand what was behind her symptoms. So I decided just to let her speak without interruption. When I spoke, I did so softly. I sat close to her and nodded my head as she talked. I probably spent twenty-five minutes with Kelly at the first consultation, despite the queue building up outside. I arranged an appointment for her the following day to continue the conversation. After that, she'd come in weekly.

As she talked, she recognized that many of her feelings were completely appropriate as she'd recently broken up with her boyfriend. She also realized she was going to bed too late, which was making her feel more exhausted and low in the mornings. As she became more aware, she started changing her lifestyle of her own accord. I didn't give Kelly what some of my colleagues would consider 'medicine'. What I gave her was time and safety. I provided a space for her to take her mask off and be listened to. And, through this, she was able to understand herself more and then make changes so that she felt better.

GET TO KNOW YOURSELF

When you give others the opportunity to become maskless, you quickly find that it becomes easier for you to drop your defences. This happened to me in a surprising way during a podcast conversation with Dr Vivek Murthy, who was Surgeon General of the US under President Obama. Although we'd never met or spoken before, we quickly formed a powerful connection. Vivek took a risk, displayed vulnerability and shared some quite personal things with me about his childhood and life journey. I reacted with non-judgement and compassion, and this brought us even closer.

A few moments later, I found myself revealing a personal story I'd been bottling up inside for years. I wasn't even consciously aware it had been bothering me. I shared with Vivek how I felt at a meeting at my publishers, a few years ago, on being told a major book retailer had declined to stock my first book because they 'already had one on the shelves by an Indian doctor'. I froze, at the time, and bit my tongue. No one else at the meeting said anything and the conversation quickly moved on. On the train home that evening, I would replay the conversation. I felt frustrated and confused. I also felt a sense of shame that I hadn't spoken up.

After the podcast conversation, which took place several years after the actual event, I journalled how I felt and discussed it with a few close confidants, fully processing the incident and moving on. Part of this moving on involved sending my publishers a calm and empathetic email, which triggered a lovely response from them about ways to stop this happening in future. My healing only came because, weeks earlier, I'd given another human being my full and focussed attention and a space in which to take off their mask. As a consequence, I was able to take off my own mask as well.

 (To hear this revealing conversation I had with Dr Vivek Murthy, go to www.drchatterjee.com/114.)

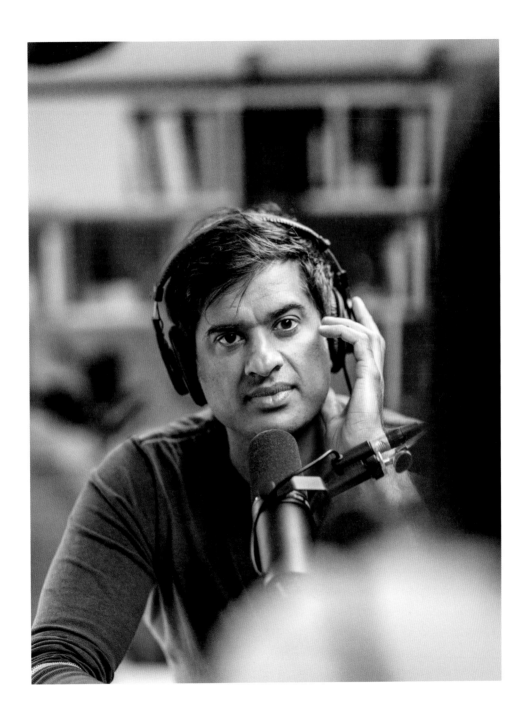

CONNECT FIRST, EDUCATE SECOND

One of the most rewarding things I do in my professional life is to teach other doctors. A big issue that routinely comes up in sessions is 'Patients don't do what I tell them.' I can always sense what the underlying problem is by the way they choose to frame this statement. The simple fact is, if you 'tell' a patient what to do, they're unlikely to do it, especially in the long term. What I advise my colleagues to do is 'connect first, educate second'. Don't rush in to give the patient the solution. First, make sure they feel heard, validated and empathized with.

This is true of all conversations, but especially those that are maskless. No one fully listens until you've connected. By connecting, you create a space for empathy and, for me, empathy is one of the most important qualities a doctor can have. In her wonderful book *Reclaiming Conversation: The Power of Talk in a Digital Age*, Sherry Turkle writes that 'empathy is not merely about giving someone information or helping them find a support group. It is about convincing another person that you are there for the duration. Empathy means staying long enough for someone to believe that you want to know how they feel, not that you want to tell them what you would do in their circumstance. Empathy requires time and emotional discipline.'

When you're listening fully, and being truly empathetic, you become humbled. You often realize that, actually, you don't know how the other person is feeling. This is why it's crucial to be attentive, patient and caring.

10 Rules for Listening

1
Be non-judgemental.

2
Be curious.

3
Practise true empathy: not 'I know how you're feeling,' but 'I don't know how you're feeling but I am here for you.'

4
Take time to really listen; don't just think about the next thing you're going to say.

5
Show them you are listening with your body language – posture, tone of voice, eye contact, not being distracted by your phone.

6
Don't try to predict where the conversation will go next.

7
Embrace silence.

8
Repeat back what they're saying in your own language.

9
Don't try to fix them or rush in to tell them what *you* would do. Instead, try asking 'How did that feel for you?' and then actively listen without interruption.

10
Have no attachment to the outcome of the conversation.

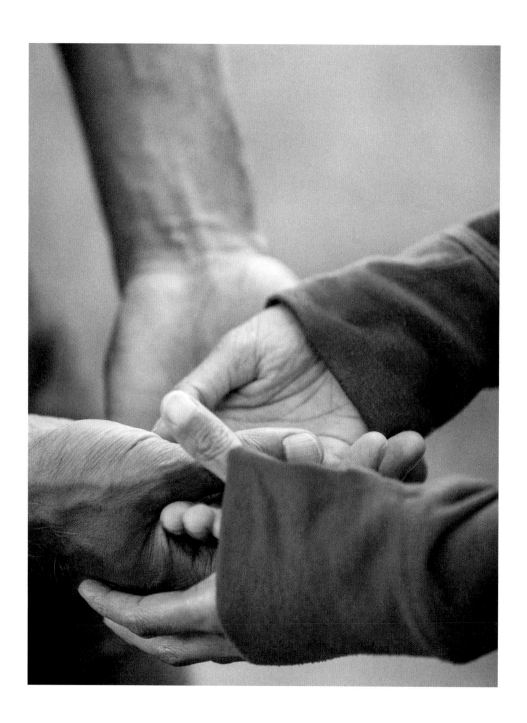

CONCLUSION

Taking off our masks is about trust, connection and love. Something powerful happens when we feel properly listened to and valued. Starting from today, I'd like you to become more aware of when you wear your masks. Learn when it's helpful to wear them and learn when it's better to go without. Make time for regular catch-ups with the people you feel close to and the people who will hear and see you. Be somebody else's miracle by creating a safe space for others to take off their masks with you. Understand that being vulnerable is your superpower. And don't be afraid. As psychologist and my friend Pippa Grange says, 'If you are constantly performing at life, you are not living life.' So, what are you waiting for? Be brave. Take off those masks and start to live.

№ 9

GO ON HOLIDAY
EVERY DAY

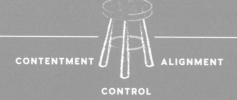

CONTENTMENT   ALIGNMENT

CONTROL

One of my friends used to work at a factory. The other day, he told me of a memory from those days that's never left him. Some of his managers had counters on their desks, literally counting the days down until their holiday. 'Only eighty-one days until I'm in Florida!' his immediate boss would say. This memory stuck with my friend, because it hinted at how unsatisfying his colleagues found their everyday lives.

If you're wishing your life away like this, desperately counting down the time until you can escape it, then you can't be happy: you're not calm, you're not aligned, and often you're the very opposite of content. When my friend told me about those factory managers, it set my mind spinning. I realized I'd never really thought before about what, exactly, a holiday is. What is it about holidays that makes them so precious? What were they getting in Florida, Spain or Sharm el Sheikh that they weren't getting at home?

WHAT IS A HOLIDAY?

Of course, there are loads of things people enjoy on their holidays: time with the family, delicious food, a drink or two, perhaps a hike or a spot of window-shopping. But all these things are available to most of us every weekend: we even get a few weeks of hot sun in the UK, if we're lucky. I believe the true joy of holidays is the sense of calmness and space they give us – the feeling that we've stepped outside our everyday life. Being away from the hassles of home, with nothing pressing scheduled, means we have time to ponder, breathe and reflect. Even on the plane on the way out to my destination, I find I'm able to get a special kind of perspective on my life. And this, I think, is what's so uniquely wonderful about that feeling of lying on the lounger by the pool with no guilt and nothing to look at but a perfect blue sky.

Holidays allow us to zoom out from our day-to-day lives in a way we often can't when we're at home. Even on a family holiday, most of us will get little moments of calm, mental stillness and reflection. Simply being in a new place and living life at a different pace make it easier to put some distance between us and our ordinary lives. Even if you feel busy trying to entertain your kids, the flavour of that busyness feels different because the background stresses of home and work have been removed.

But we don't have to actually go anywhere to have this experience. We can treat ourselves to a holiday every day by finding a small, protected space to gain some mental stillness, perspective and reflection. One of the best ways to do this is with a daily practice of solitude. Solitude isn't about being lonely, it's the positive, intentional practice of being by yourself. The ability to enjoy your own company is essential for happiness. For myself, I'd go so far as to say that taking a daily holiday is a non-negotiable. On the days I don't, I'm noticeably less happy.

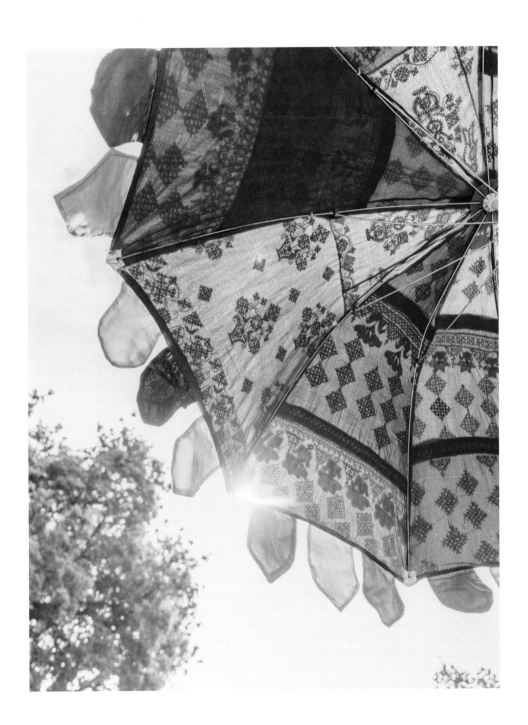

SOLITUDE'S ASTONISHING GIFT

What does solitude give us that's so valuable? Whether we're getting it on a sun-lounger on holiday or a yoga mat on our kitchen floor, one of its great gifts is reflection. Solitude enables us to calmly and mindfully survey our life and, in doing so, strengthen our Core Happiness by building our sense of contentment and control and moving us back into alignment. It helps us get in touch with our innermost feelings, to process our anxieties, and offers the possibility of a fresh perspective. We become more in tune with ourselves and, in turn, with the world around us.

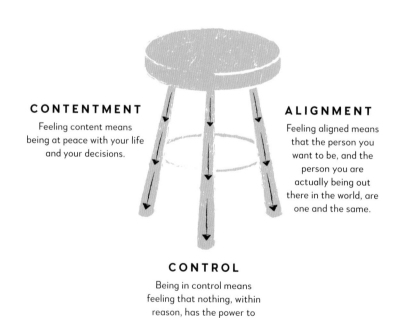

CONTENTMENT
Feeling content means being at peace with your life and your decisions.

ALIGNMENT
Feeling aligned means that the person you want to be, and the person you are actually being out there in the world, are one and the same.

CONTROL
Being in control means feeling that nothing, within reason, has the power to overwhelm you.

Despite its enormous benefits, many of my patients find solitude and reflection difficult. While they'd happily while away a week by the hotel pool, when they get home they find ten minutes of mindful me-time all but impossible. This is partly down to our fast-paced culture and the Want Brain world that surrounds us with its distractions and temptations. Most people who struggle this way are simply not used to sitting with their own thoughts. But if we're serious about getting happier, we must get serious about solitude and reflection.

As much as we might sometimes want to, we can't escape ourselves. So, our only option is to get to know ourselves. Reflection enables us to do this and it is crucial if we want to achieve alignment. Reflection allows us to see who we are and where we are in our journey of becoming who we aspire to be. If there's a foggy pane of glass between ourselves and our happiness, reflection starts to clean it. It helps us tap into our innate wisdom.

This time alone also allows us to hear the signals our body is trying to send us. When I was a junior doctor, I remember being taught about early warning signs. By taking regular measurements of key parameters like our breathing rate, heart rate and temperature, I learned that we could predict which patients were going to get seriously ill hours in advance of it happening. By spotting when their parameters were moving in that direction, we could get involved straight away and prevent it. Going on a daily holiday allows us to tune into our own early warning systems and detect when our bodies are giving out subtle signs that they might be struggling in some way. I know when my stress load is building because I feel it in a particular place beneath my right shoulder. This occasional discomfort has been going on for many years but, incredibly, I've only just become aware of it, because of my daily holiday practice. I now use it as an early warning that tells me that my stress load is going up. I know that if I don't do something, I may end up snapping at the kids or getting wound up on social media. Only because I've taken the time to step out of my life every day do I have the ability to register and remedy the problem.

The Benefits of Taking a Daily Holiday

Taking a daily holiday helps us to:

- Reflect on our lives

- Gain a new perspective on day-to-day problems

- Access mental stillness

- Increase awareness of our innermost emotions
  and hear the signals our body is sending us

- Change the pace of our day

- Reduce anxiety

- Improve our sense of calm

- Understand that we are worth taking care of

MOVING HOLIDAYS

For many of us, movement is the easiest way to take a daily holiday and access some mental stillness. And, of course, we do tend to move our bodies more when we're actually away, whether we're swimming in the pool, exploring a new city or enjoying long walks in nature. Movement can be particularly powerful when our minds have become overactive or we feel stuck in a spiral of negative thoughts.

There are many different ways to access mental stillness while moving. Buddhists have an ancient practice of walking meditation. There's something hypnotic about the repetition of motion, with one foot in front of the other, that helps us switch off the 'thinking' part of the brain and tune into something calmer and more creative. Multiple studies have shown how walking can help lift depression and boost mental health, especially if it's out in nature. My brother takes his own daily holiday with either a thirty-minute run or walk. When he comes back, he tells me his problems seem that bit smaller and issues that he felt he couldn't solve before can feel eminently solvable.

Another friend of mine loves to practise Vipassana meditation as he runs. He starts concentrating on his breath, then slowly moves his attention from the crown of his head all the way down his body to the tips of his toes and slowly back up again. It's an intensive form of self-workout that brilliantly combines physical and mental wellbeing.

But it's really not necessary to over-complicate this with prescriptive rules. Any form of movement that you enjoy doing will suffice. Even a ten-minute walk around the block in a city can provide incredible benefits for body and mind. All you are looking for is something that helps you step outside the noise of your day-to-day life and, for a short period of time, allows you to feel calm, still and to reflect.

Regular moving is especially important for those of us with sedentary jobs. The fact is, our minds and bodies are simply not designed to be so physically passive. Much of our work these days is carried out by our brains. Yet, for tens of thousands of years, it would have been physical: digging for tubers in the hard-packed ground, building shelters, walking for hours to a hunt.

Examples of moving daily holidays include:

- Walking

- Running

- Yoga

- Swimming

- Cycling

(All of the above have benefits, but I do think, in our constantly connected, fast-paced world, that there is something uniquely special about swimming. Being submersed under water allows us to get away from technology and turn down the volume of daily life like nothing else.)

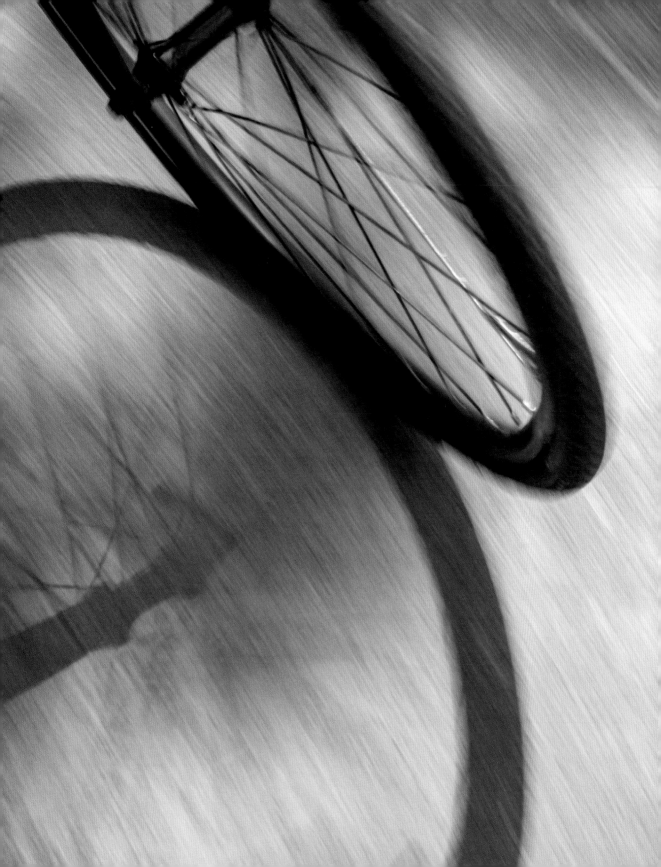

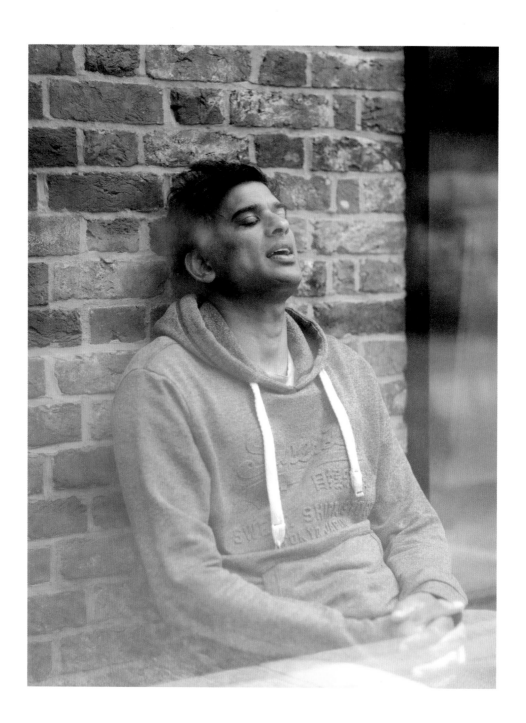

SITTING STILLNESS

As important as movement is, it's crucial that you do not come to rely on it as your only practice of solitude. If you do, you may miss out on some of the incredible benefits that sitting practices can offer us. Practices such as meditation, journalling or breathwork can sometimes help us access and unlock different emotions than those unlocked by moving ones.

This is exactly what happened with one of my patients, 58-year-old Miranda. She would go running or walking every day and told me that this was her meditation. She told me that sitting practices were not for her – she was much better suited to moving ones, which she really enjoyed. I explained that while running was certainly meditative for her, it was not a substitute for a sitting practice of stillness. Miranda was a people-pleaser. She kept herself busy helping others, but this affected her sleep and her ability to switch off. People around her thought she was super-happy, but I suspected her inability to sit quietly with her thoughts was a sign that something deeper was affecting her wellbeing.

I convinced Miranda that it was worth experimenting with ten minutes of journalling each day to see if she gained a different kind of perspective on life compared to when she was running. Within a week, she'd started to articulate thoughts about a relationship with a friend that had turned sour twenty years earlier.

Over the course of that year, Miranda started the process of repairing previous fractured relationships. She called up her old friend and they met up. She also started the process of repairing her broken relationship with her brother. All of this made her feel substantially calmer, more content and aligned. She'd have never got there through running alone. This is why I agree with the Vietnamese Buddhist monk Thich Nhat Hanh, who once gave the brilliant instruction, 'Don't just do something, sit there.'

Miranda had kept herself busy by *doing*. From the outside, her life looked great – she enjoyed her job and was proactive about taking care of her health. But, in reality, her busyness, although seemingly 'healthy', was actually her method of running away from deeper emotions that her mind had kept locked away. A sitting practice of solitude – in Miranda's case, journalling – helped her get to know herself in a way that walking and running did not.

This type of scenario is not unique to Miranda. Twenty-first-century living is busy and fast-paced and many of us live in a chronic state of overwhelm. Even when we try to switch off and press pause, we still look for more things to do. We forget that we are human beings. We need less *doing* and more *being*. This is something that a lot of us find challenging, but it is well worth persevering with, as the benefits can be transformative.

"

If there's a foggy
pane of glass between
ourselves and our
happiness, reflection
starts to clean it.

"

MAKE STILLNESS A SUPERPOWER

There's another crucial reason why it's important to be able to access stillness and solitude without having to rely on movement. And that is freedom. If you are only able to gain perspective on your life and access mental stillness when moving, you leave yourself in a vulnerable position. You are reliant on a functional, injury-free body to access your solitude and stillness. What would happen if you were to sprain your ankle and were unable to walk? What if you were to twist your knee and were unable to run? These are common scenarios that I've seen frequently cause problems. I know many patients and have friends who become anxious, frustrated and depressed when they're unable to train due to injury.

One of my patients, 54-year-old Wendy, loved to take a daily holiday with a walk in nature. It helped her relax, switch off from life and reflect. But a few years back she started to suffer with pain in the soles of her feet and was unable to walk for months. She really struggled, as she had no other method to switch off and reflect and quickly spiralled into mental turmoil. It was only when I encouraged her to start a daily practice of meditation that she began to regain a sense of control within her life and feel calm and content.

This same principle of freedom also applies to external devices. Only being able to switch off when you have your phone and earbuds to hand makes you a prisoner. I know many people who are so reliant on their headphones when they are out running or walking that if their headphones don't work for any reason or their phone runs out of battery they experience low-grade anxiety and end up feeling stressed, frustrated and annoyed. What should be a relaxing and restorative 'daily holiday' quickly turns into a stress-inducing nightmare. Has that ever happened to you?

Over time, I want you to develop the skill of being able to take a daily holiday without the need for anything apart from yourself. This is the ultimate freedom and, when you are able to do this, you massively strengthen all three legs of the Core Happiness stool. You feel content, profoundly in control of your life and much more aligned. I am not saying for one minute that this is easy. Just as running a marathon takes months of regular practice, developing the skill to sit in silence and alone with your thoughts also takes time and patience. Please don't let that put you off. You don't want to hack and fast-track this process. The process itself is where you'll find the gold.

As you practise, you will learn more and more about yourself. What do you find difficult? When do you get distracted? What are you reliant on to switch off and press pause? Where does your mind go when you have no distractions? Learning this is crucial and is rewarding in and of itself. You cannot learn about these things from reading this book or any other book. You can only learn them through experience.

It's only in the past year or two that I have felt able to access mental stillness at any time without the need for any external help, and I have been practising for a while. I no longer need a meditation app in order to meditate, but sometimes I choose to use one. I love to go for long walks and listen to podcasts or music, but I am equally content going without.

The aim of this book is to help you become the architect of your own health and happiness. As a society, we are becoming more and more conditioned to needing things, objects and apps in order for us to feel calm and content. If you are unable to sit in silence with your own thoughts, your happiness is always going to be dependent on other things. As the philosopher Blaise Pascal wrote, 'All of humanity's problems stem from the inability to sit quietly in a room alone.' Being able to access stillness any time, anywhere, will become your superpower.

CASE STUDY

Sali was a 31-year-old digital marketer, working in the beauty industry, who came to see me with troublesome gut symptoms. She'd have to open her bowels several times per day, which was negatively impacting her work and social life. Previous doctors had put this down to IBS and gave her a variety of different medications which, unfortunately, didn't help her. Her unmanaged symptoms were affecting how Sali felt about herself and she'd often take it out on her husband, which was starting to affect their relationship.

Over the course of my career, I have found that stress is a major trigger for gut symptoms, even more so than diet. I wasn't surprised to find that Sali was always living around her stress threshold, working from home with two children and a husband who also worked from home. Time was always scarce and she felt guilty when she wasn't doing something. She never gave herself time to herself.

I told Sali a daily holiday would be tremendously helpful to her. She told me running had once been a passion but now she didn't really have time to do it 'properly'. In her head, only one-hour runs counted and she felt guilty about taking that much time out.

I explained that running for twenty or thirty minutes would still be beneficial, not least for her mental health. It would allow her to step outside her life and reflect. I explained that this form of 'holiday' would also enable her to be more productive when she got back to work.

Four weeks later, Sali told me she was feeling more like herself, and she could now clearly see that she was working too hard. She'd also noticed a significant improvement in her gut symptoms. She was managing to run three times a week and, on the days she did, she felt less anxious, less stressed and slept better.

I explained to her that she needed a holiday from her life every day, not just three times a week. If she didn't want to run on the other days, she could try other forms of movement or, perhaps, a sitting practice of stillness. She decided to start with daily ten-minute yoga flows. Six months later, after further improvements, I asked her to add in five minutes of meditation each day. This allowed her to really listen to her body and tune into her mind in a completely different way to running and yoga. Twelve months later, she had no gut symptoms at all.

How to Take Your Daily Holiday

Everyone's daily holiday will be unique to them. Experiment with different options and see what works for you and your lifestyle. You can switch it up from day to day as your needs and daily timetable changes.

The crucial component of this practice is that it allows you time to turn your thoughts inward and enable you to reflect on your life. What we're looking for is time to step outside our lives and gain solitude and perspective.

Use the following principles to guide you. You don't need to stick to them all, but the more you manage the better:

- Something you do alone

- Something that brings you into the present moment

- Something that doesn't rely on a smartphone

- Something that is done in complete silence

Many people find moving holidays much easier to begin with. Perhaps you currently go for daily walks with your headphones on. This is fantastic. Now see if, a couple of times per week, you can go without your earbuds on and immerse yourself in silence or the sound of your breathing. The key is to be kind to yourself. This is not a competition or a race, it's a lifelong practice. All we're looking for is small amounts of progress.

Over time, I want you to work up to incorporating a form of sitting stillness into your life. In my experience, the best ways to do this are with breathwork, journalling or meditation.

For me, I have a selection of practices from which I take my daily holiday. My moving practice will be either a walk, a run, a swim or, occasionally, a bike ride. My sitting practices will be meditation, breathwork or journalling. Feel free to create your own practices if you feel there is something more suitable to you and your life.

JOURNALLING

Many incredible figures throughout history have advocated the benefits of journalling. The Stoic philosophers Marcus Aurelius and slave turned teacher Seneca understood how powerful and useful this is as a daily practice. For the Stoic thinkers, the daily journal wasn't simply a diary, it was the building block on which their entire philosophy of life was built.

From my perspective, journalling is incredible because it's one of those habits that hits all three legs of the Core Happiness stool. Getting your thoughts out of your head and on to the page creates valuable space between you and your emotions, which helps you feel both calmer and more in control. It's an especially useful practice for alignment. Journalling allows you to have a conversation with yourself. Within days, you'll find you've got to know yourself better, and the benefits will only compound further over time. Some days, you'll have real breakthroughs; other days, you might feel you're simply going through the process. But, bit by bit, you'll be able to see more clearly where you're moving out of alignment and develop the wisdom to know how to correct your course. I find the repetition of daily journalling is, in itself, deeply therapeutic.

There are many different ways of keeping a journal. You could keep a traditional long-form diary or simply write down three words that describe how you're feeling in the moment. Some people like to copy out an inspirational quote. Whatever you choose to do, the act of physically writing your journal out in longhand is crucial. It helps to imprint the ideas into your subconscious in a way that just thinking about them or typing them into your phone doesn't.

 (To read more about different journalling practices, go to drchatterjee.com/journalling. And to listen to the podcast conversation I had with the neuroscientist Dr Tara Swart about the power of journalling, visit www.drchatterjee.com/58.)

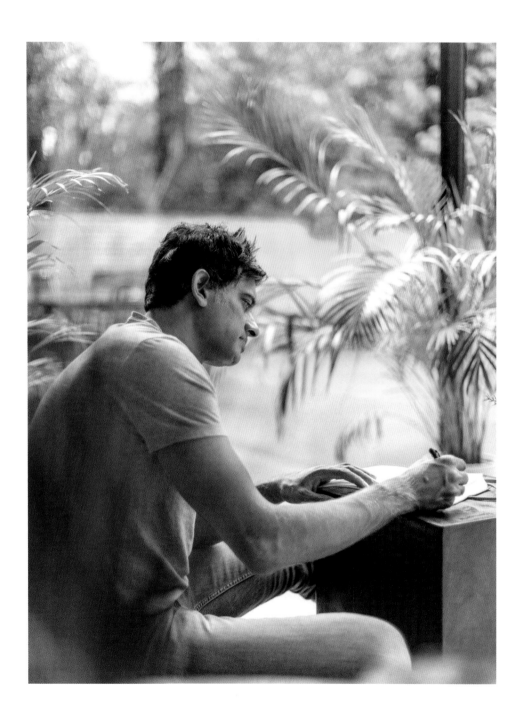

BREATHWORK

Consciously paying attention to your breath is a simple yet massively underrated practice for health and happiness. Changing your breathing changes your biology and your state of mind. By breathing through your nose rather than your mouth, from your abdomen instead of solely from your chest, and by making your out-breath longer than your in-breath, you intentionally manipulate your body's stress response. You send signals to your brain that tell it you're safe. This strengthens Core Happiness by making you calmer and more in control. It also helps us get to know ourselves, which in turn makes it easier for us to be aligned. And it improves health by moving your body out of its damaging stress state.

For people who suffer with anxiety and are trapped in a cycle of negative thinking, breathwork can be transformative. Often, we unsuccessfully try to use the mind to solve the mind's problems. This sounds reasonable and logical, but it can actually be very hard to fix the mind with the mind. The mind is taking in signals from the world around it. Many of these signals are channelled through the body. Intentionally changing the body's signals is a powerful hack that goes deep into the mind.

Breathwork helps calm the emotional turbulence we feel inside us. It helps us become more resilient to stress and tune in to our inner thoughts and emotions. Taking a daily holiday with an intentional practice of breathwork can be seriously life-changing. In many respects, the way you breathe determines the way you live. It empowers us by giving us a choice: do we want to allow stress to be in charge of us, or do we want to be in charge of stress?

 (To help you choose a breathwork practice that suits you, visit drchatterjee.com/breathing and if you want to learn more about the life-changing benefits of breathwork for physical and mental health, you can access podcast conversations I have had with James Nestor, Patrick McKeown and Brian MacKenzie at drchatterjee.com/breathwork.)

"

We are so busy
trying to do more,
be more and get
more, that we forget
about the pleasure
of simply being.

—

"

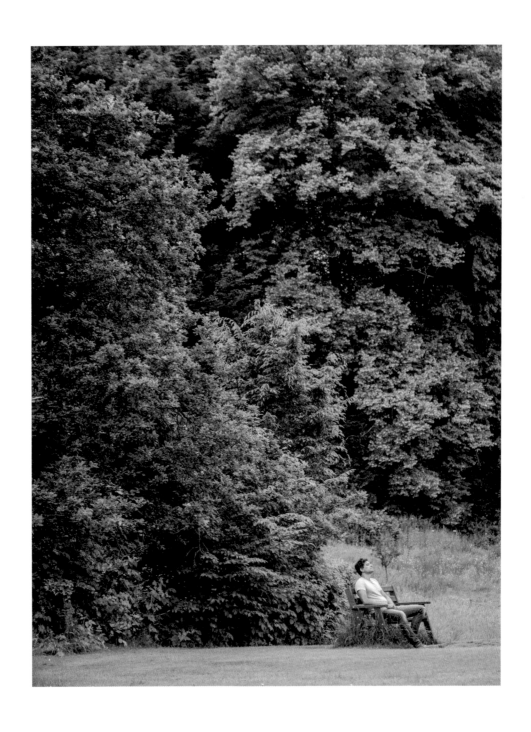

MEDITATION

Meditation is one of the most effective forms of daily holiday that exist. When practiced regularly, it offers benefits that very few other practices can match and has powerful effects on our body and mind. It has been shown to reduce stress, improve focus and enhance sleep. It enables us to gain a unique perspective on our lives, increasing self-awareness and our capacity to be fully present. It's even been shown to reduce negative emotions, increase creativity and reduce our perception of pain.

Despite these incredible benefits, many of us struggle to even start a regular meditation practice. We're so used to filling up our time with busyness that taking a pause and just being seems like a revolutionary, almost crazy act. Many people feel they don't have time for meditation, without realizing that it actually gives back more time than it uses. The influential author and historian Yuval Noah Harari makes time to meditate for a full two hours every day and puts his ability to write incredible books such as the multi-million global bestseller *Sapiens* down to this daily practice.

Contrary to popular belief, meditation is not about switching off your mind. It is about making friends with it. It's about being fully present to *all* the thoughts that pop up and being non-judgmental about them. This helps us be the observer of our thoughts and feelings, rather than the victim of them, which helps us feel calm and in control. The benefits of meditation are mostly seen outside of the practice itself. On days that you meditate, you'll find that later in the day you're less reactive and less prone to getting stressed. You'll feel calmer, more present and have a much clearer perspective on your life.

(To help you choose a meditation practice that suits you and your life, visit drchatterjee.com/meditation, and to listen to my podcast conversation with renowned meditation teacher Light Watkins, visit www.drchatterjee.com/23.)

FROM ROUTINE TO RITUAL

When you first start a daily holiday practice, it will feel like something you do as a routine. But once it begins to work its magic on you, it'll start to feel less like a routine and more like a ritual. The difference between them lies in your attitude and intention. A routine is something you do regularly, like taking out the bins. But a ritual is enveloped in meaning. It's a daily act of self-love, your excuse to care about yourself, to remove yourself from the pressures of the world and to remind yourself that you are of supreme value. It's a practice that's sacred to you and that leaves a noticeable emotional hole when you don't do it.

Your ritual will be unique to you. It can be one single practice, or a sequence of them. My morning routine starts with making the bed. This might sound like nothing, but it has a profound impact on how I feel about myself. It allows me to feel that I've accomplished the first task of the day with order and care. This feeling of control over disorder strengthens my Core Happiness. I then do my '3 M morning routine', which I first wrote about in my second book, *The Stress Solution*, and which has always been popular with my readers. These 3 Ms consist of Mindfulness, Movement and Mindset. For me, this looks like five minutes of breathwork, then ten minutes of meditation, followed by a quick five-minute workout while my coffee is brewing. I then drink my coffee while reading a book I find uplifting and energizing. All of this takes just twenty minutes or so, but it reprograms my mind, moving it into a state of calmness and wellbeing. When it is done, I feel like my inner life and my outer behaviour are matching up more precisely: I've become better aligned.

If it helps, you can make your practice feel more ritualistic by taking a few seconds before you start to acknowledge that this is you stepping out of your external world and deciding to devote some precious time to your internal world. This may be three deep breaths just before you step outside for your daily walk. It might be intentionally closing your laptop or powering down your phone before doing some yoga. It might be lighting a candle and meditating in a special place in your home where you can sit for a short while in silence. Or you might simply sit alone in a clean space with a cup of coffee and focus deeply on the experience of enjoying the drink.

It's a daily act of self-love, your excuse to care about yourself, to remove yourself from the pressures of the world and to remind yourself that you are of supreme value.

 (To watch a video of me speaking in detail about my morning routine, go to drchatterjee.com/morningroutine.)

CONCLUSION

You don't need to wait for that one week a year when you jump on an aeroplane to feel good. You can take a holiday from your life any time you like. And you should. Doing so on a daily basis will give you a new, positive perspective on your life and help you be more in tune with your body. You'll start to become more aware of yourself and how you interact with the world around you. You'll feel more in control, calmer and more aligned. Your daily holiday is like a session in the muscle gym for your Core Happiness. And the best thing about it is it always feels great.

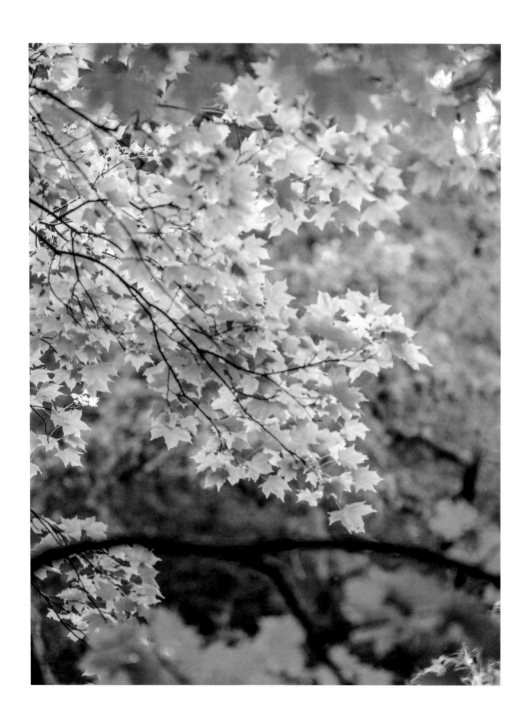

Nº· 10

GIVE YOURSELF AWAY

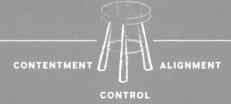

CONTENTMENT   ALIGNMENT

CONTROL

So far, every chapter of this book has been me-focused. This might be surprising, but I make no apologies for it. I'm a firm believer in the principle that, as adults, each one of us is ultimately responsible for our own alignment, contentment and sense of being in control. Nobody can strengthen our Core Happiness for us, just as, outside our duties as parents and friends, we can't do all that much about the Core Happiness of others. But this doesn't mean it's a good idea to be wholly inward-looking.

On the contrary, the research on this is clear and overwhelming: people who are other-focused are happier. Study after study has shown this. Those who give more money to charities are happier than those who give less, just as those who donate their time as volunteers are happier. The psychologist Dr Elizabeth Dunn led a study in which people were given money to spend on treating themselves or treating someone else. Afterwards, their moods were assessed. The people who were told to do something nice for others were significantly happier than those who spent the cash on themselves. People struggling with alcohol addiction who focus on being of service to others are more likely to stay sober than those who don't. An incredible 94 per cent of alcoholics who helped other alcoholics experienced lower levels of depression.

"

The individualist focus on the self can cause us to suffer.

—

"

WIRED TO GIVE

Looking outwards has powerful positive effects because we're wired to connect with others. As a tribal species, we're wired to thrive when we feel we're being of service to the people around us. We're literally built for social connection. We have special touch receptors in the skin of our forearms and upper back that are designed to respond only to being stroked. When they're activated, messages are sent to the brain that lower levels of the stress hormone cortisol. We're born with an almost magical ability to pick up on what others are feeling through tone of voice, body language, micro-expressions and even smell, so we can figure out what they're feeling and know if they need help.

Yet Want Brain cultures are individualistic. We live in nuclear families, rather than the extended families we evolved in. We often set up home many miles away from where we were born and where our support networks are based. We're encouraged to see ourselves not as members of connected communities but as isolated beings. We're bombarded with messages about how we can all improve our own lives and, in some ways, this is a good thing: individualism is based on the precious value of the individual, and this idea gave us the concept of human rights. But, in other ways, the individualist focus on the self can cause us to suffer. It makes us prone to neglect the parts of us that naturally yearn to give ourselves away to others.

WHAT RELIGIONS KNOW

It's only recently that humans started looking to scientists for the key to happiness. For the vast majority of human history, we'd have looked instead to spiritual leaders for this kind of help. The religions these wise elders represented were extremely ancient – and often extremely wise. I was raised in a Hindu family that originated in Kolkata, India. The big celebration of our year is a multi-day event called Durga Puja. I remember going along as a child and, yes, there were loads of mantras, prayers and rituals, but there was also a real sense of community and connection. At the end of each ceremony, it was customary for everyone to be fed. Volunteers were required to make this happen. One year I got roped into serving food. Initially, I didn't want to help and was upset that I wasn't allowed to continue playing with my friends. But afterwards, I remember feeling absolutely fantastic.

The Want Brain often tries to persuade us not to surrender ourselves for a greater good. It says, 'What's in it for me?' But religions have known for thousands of years that it's crucial to push past these all-too-natural feelings. Doing things for others powerfully strengthens all three legs of the Core Happiness stool. We feel content, in control and much more aligned as, deep down, we all want to be the kind of person that helps others.

It's no coincidence that *all* religions have the idea of giving yourself away, in some form or other, at their core. In the secular, scientific world, we're only just starting to catch up with how fundamental this is to our psychological wellbeing. We now know that giving ourselves away can have a powerful impact on our mood and reduce symptoms of depression. When we're feeling down, the quickest and most effective way of building happiness is by looking outwards.

Volunteering has been found to boost mood, reduce stress and help us live longer. Amazingly, it even stretches our perception of time, making us feel less time poor and stressed. As we learned in Chapter 4, this can have incredible benefits for Core Happiness. This is a crucial point to remember, as the fast pace of twenty-first-century life results in many of us feeling as if we are too busy to give ourselves away.

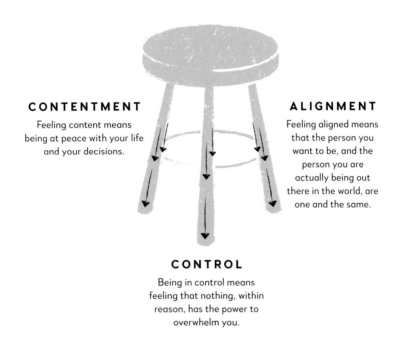

CONTENTMENT

Feeling content means being at peace with your life and your decisions.

ALIGNMENT

Feeling aligned means that the person you want to be, and the person you are actually being out there in the world, are one and the same.

CONTROL

Being in control means feeling that nothing, within reason, has the power to overwhelm you.

How did you feel, in your heart and soul, the last time you gave yourself away?

GRATITUDE AND FORGIVENESS

There's a lot more to giving yourself away than just physically being there for other people. Being able to surrender our selfish thought patterns is also an essential ingredient for happiness. When we become overly me-focused, we tend to forget to feel grateful for the parts of our life that are actually good. We also fail to forgive people who we come into conflict with. Being thankful for what we have, and actively and intentionally practising forgiveness, are common spiritual practices for a simple reason – they work.

They make our relationships stronger, which makes our social world safer, and this makes us feel more in control. They make us feel more content and at peace with the world, and they also make us more aligned with who we want to be: nobody feels good about themselves when they're continually ungrateful and hold on to grudges. A wealth of modern research backs up what religions have known for millennia. Holding on to jealousy, anger and envy has been found to put our mind and body into stress state. It signals to our brain that we're in an unsafe space, which can trigger more stress and a spiral down into depression. Forgiveness reverses this process, sending us on an upward spiral towards happiness.

Gratitude has also been proven to have a powerful effect on happiness. Humans are primed for the negative. This is because our brains evolved in dangerous times. Back in the Stone Age, we'd benefit from being hyper-alert to any event in our lives that might threaten to hurt us. Today, we live lives that are immeasurably safer than they once were, yet our brains are still programmed for that ancient environment. Psychologists find that we take in roughly nine bits of negative information for every positive bit. This is bad news for Core Happiness. It gives us a distorted, overly anxious view of the world, and can make us feel out of control and discontented.

Gratitude is the cure for negativity. It's been shown to lower anxiety, improve sleep, reduce symptoms of depression and have a positive effect on relationships, empathy and self-esteem. It has also been shown to improve blood pressure and our perception of pain. Gratitude is a social emotion that reminds us how supported and safe we are and connects us to the people around us. Every year the University of Chicago psychologist Professor Nicholas Epley asks his students to write a letter of gratitude to someone who's done something meaningful for them who they've not yet had the chance to thank. Before they send the letter, they're asked to predict how both they and the recipient of the letter will feel when it's sent. Epley finds they not only significantly underestimate how happy the recipient will feel, they also underestimate how happy they themselves will become.

Either as a stand-alone practice, or combined with journalling, intentionally feeling gratitude every day is virtually a non-negotiable for happiness. It has powerful effects on our physical health and mental wellbeing and, best of all, it's completely free. It lowers anxiety and brings us into alignment. It also increases our sense of control, because it moves us out of ruminating about the past or worrying about the future and into the present.

As an added bonus, practising gratitude is even thought to make us more able to experience flow state (see page 102).

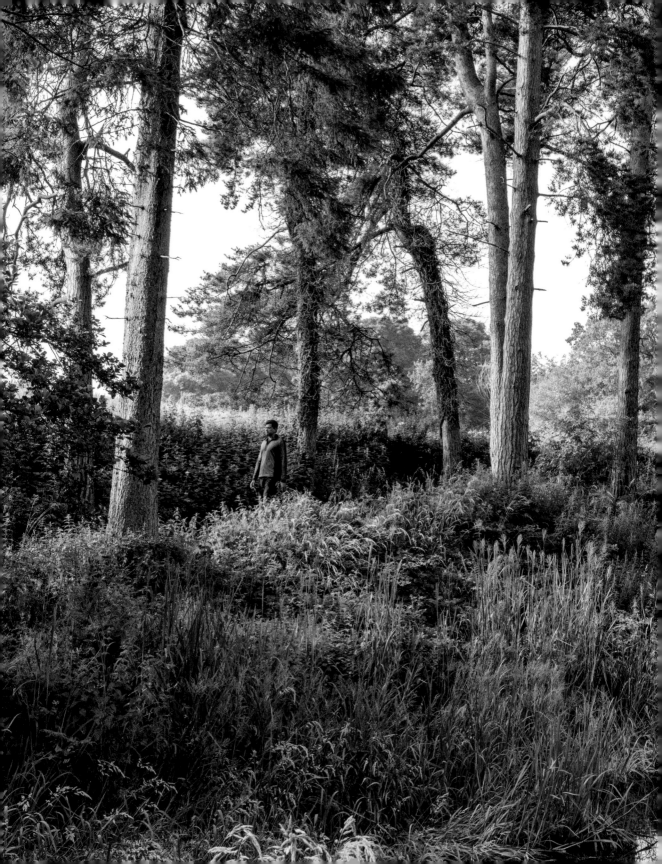

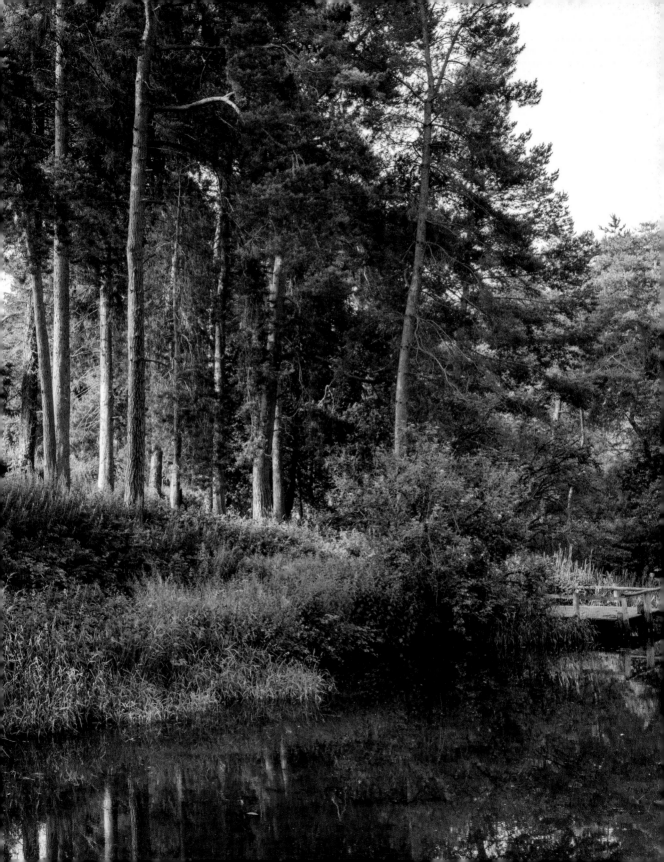

Practise Gratitude

Gratitude is an emotion that connects you to your social world. I'd like you to pick a gratitude habit that really speaks to you and do it regularly. Here are some options to get you started:

- Write a Gratitude Letter to someone once a week. Write down things they have done for you in the past and express your thanks. Be as specific as you can. For example, you could say thank you to someone who helped you move flats when you were in your twenties. Or a friend who helped you prepare for a job interview. I would encourage you to send the letter but, even if you don't, the act of simply writing it will provide you with most of the benefits.

- Write down in your journal three to five things you are grateful for in your life each day. You could start each day with this practice or, perhaps, do it last thing at night to help you switch off and relax. Over time, you can supercharge its effectiveness by making it more specific and detailed. For each thing you are grateful for, you could start off with a simple thought and then see if you can write a full paragraph on it.

- Around the dinner table with your friends and family, take it in turns to share three things you are grateful for. Remember, be as specific as you can and try to make them different each day.

- In a moment of stress or anxiety, take a pause and just shift your attention to something you are grateful for in your life. Anything, no matter how simple, will start to make you feel more aligned, content and in control.

The more you practise gratitude, the easier it becomes and the more you train your mind to be grateful in all aspects of your life. It doesn't take much time and is completely free. But it only works if you do it. What are you waiting for?

HOW RELIGION BUILDS CORE HAPPINESS

Research shows us that people who engage in religious practices are happier than those who don't. In this chapter, we've explored how religion compels people to give themselves away by practising forgiveness, gratitude and by giving the gift of their time. But these are not the only ways religion builds Core Happiness. I learned this during the years I spent as a GP in Oldham, treating patients from some of the UK's most deprived socio-economic groups. Many were first-generation immigrants whose lives were exhausting and tough. They were living far away from the support networks of home, not earning much money and often doing arduous and repetitive jobs where they were not valued or respected.

However, a lot of them were happy regardless of their struggles, because they had a strong connection to their faith. The support that religion gave them was brought home to me when I saw a young couple whose baby had recently died from cot death. It was their first child. When they came in, I treated them with tenderness and empathy. In a soft and compassionate voice, I asked them how they were. They told me it was God's will for this to happen, so there had to be a reason. Initially, I was a little shocked to hear this. But as I thought about it more, I came to realize this was their faith holding them up. Their strong belief in religion was carrying them through what is arguably one of the most painful experiences it's possible to have.

Religion gave this couple an incredibly powerful sense of control. They believed there was order, justice and stability in the universe. Everything that happened was ordained by God, who was by definition good. Religion also directly strengthens the other two legs of the Core Happiness stool. It provides a powerful toolbox for maximizing contentment. If we're feeling regretful or ruminative, we can meditate, pray or take comfort in the Scriptures. Finally, of course, it gives us a programme for inner and outer alignment. It tells us what kind of person we should strive to be, then offers help in the form of sacred texts and religious advisers, whether they're priests, rabbis or imams. This, I believe, is why religion has been so successful and popular for thousands of years. It's evolved to keep our Core Happiness stool strong and upright – in even the very worst of situations.

Of course, we don't need to be religious to gain these benefits. This book aims to provide you with a framework that you can apply in your own life, whether you choose to follow a religion or not.

HAVE WE GOT IT WRONG AS DOCTORS?

Almost all the advice that doctors like myself give their patients involves doing things in isolation. We tell them to change their diet, go to the gym, take this or that medication. We're trained to view the sick as individuals, rather than parts of a collective whole. But humans are herd animals. We do better in groups. Could this mean that we also heal better in groups?

Powerful evidence that this might be the case comes from an inspiring GP based in Somerset. In 2013, Dr Helen Kingston was moved to launch the Compassionate Frome Project after noticing that many of her patients felt they were being treated as little more than their symptoms. She began connecting patients into community groups, whether they be choirs, writing workshops, lunch clubs or talking cafés, where people with similar symptoms could get together and chat.

Incredibly, following the project's launch, emergency admissions at Frome's hospital went down by 15 per cent. Elsewhere in Somerset, admissions rocketed by 30 per cent. As Dr Julian Abel, a retired consultant in palliative care, said, 'No other interventions on record have reduced emergency admissions across a population.' What was it, ultimately, that led to these incredible results? Simple. The people of Frome gave themselves away to each other.

 (To listen to a powerful conversation I had with Dr Julian Abel on my podcast about these incredible findings and the healing power of compassion, visit www.drchatterjee.com/138.)

CASE STUDY

Over the past few years, there's been a growing interest in what's been termed 'social prescribing'. This is when we ask a patient to engage in activities with others, like cookery classes, book clubs, gardening, parkrun or volunteering. The early indications are that the physical and mental health benefits of social prescribing are huge.

A few years ago, I started seeing a patient who said she didn't want to live. Tanesha was twenty-three and had recently graduated from university with a great degree. Her future looked bright, but she felt low, indifferent and had very little motivation to do anything. On the rare occasions she experienced pleasure, it always seemed short-lived. Inevitably, she found solace in Junk Happiness, drinking wine to numb her pain and binge-watching reality television and YouTube videos.

As I got to know her better, I noticed that she rarely mentioned her family, friends or loved ones. Her parents and brothers lived in Birmingham, and she hadn't stayed in touch with any of her university friends. One of the rare times I saw Tanesha truly laugh was when I suggested that she try to lift her mood by going to parkrun. 'You don't need to run,' I said. 'You can just volunteer.' Rather reluctantly, she agreed to give it a go.

On the first Saturday, she helped put the cones up, then went to work marshalling a corner of the race, making sure people were heading in the right direction. She didn't say much, in terms of words of support for the runners, as she felt a little bit self-conscious and out of place. But over the coming weeks, as Tanesha began to feel more at ease, she started encouraging others, shouting, 'You can do it!' and 'Just one kilometre to go!' When she came back after a week off, one of the runners shouted out to her as he ran past her, 'We missed you last week, Tanesha! Good to see you back.' To her utter surprise, she felt a lump in her throat. Tears of joy began to well in her eyes.

To say volunteering changed Tanesha's life is an understatement. In a matter of months, she'd gone from having occasional suicidal thoughts to being completely clear of depression. This was an improvement that no amount of medication or talking therapy could ever hope to match. Her problem wasn't a serotonin deficiency – it was a feeling-needed deficiency. The CEO of parkrun once told me on my podcast that parkrun is actually a 'social intervention masquerading as a running event'. I couldn't put it better myself.

 (To listen to the podcast conversation I had with Nick Pearson, the CEO of parkrun, visit www.drchatterjee.com/42.)

THE KINDNESS WAVE

It's incredible, but true: research suggests that practising kindness may have more of an effect on health and happiness than diet and exercise. Acts of kindness send a signal to your brain that life is great. This switches it out of unhealthy stress state and into thrive state. One study in Japan found that when people simply take the time to count their own acts of kindness every week, they become happier. Another found that the more kind acts you carry out, the happier you become. It didn't matter whether these acts of kindness were for loved ones or complete strangers, the effects on happiness were the same.

But perhaps the most magical quality of kindness is the way it ripples out into the world. When I spoke to Dr David Hamilton – a brilliant expert on interactions between the mind and the body – he told me that 'given the average amount of interconnectedness we have with others and the amount of social interactions we have in any given day, you'd probably find the person you just helped would be kinder to five more people throughout the rest of the day. Those five people will probably be kinder to five more people, and each of those five people will be kinder to five more people.'

It's reasonable to conclude, then, that one single small act of kindness on any given day will help spread kindness to over a hundred people. When you decide to give yourself away with a simple act of kindness, you're sending a beautiful wave of happiness that will travel far into the world and deep into hearts.

 (To listen to the podcast conversation I had with Dr David Hamilton about the healing power of kindness, visit www.drchatterjee.com/104.)

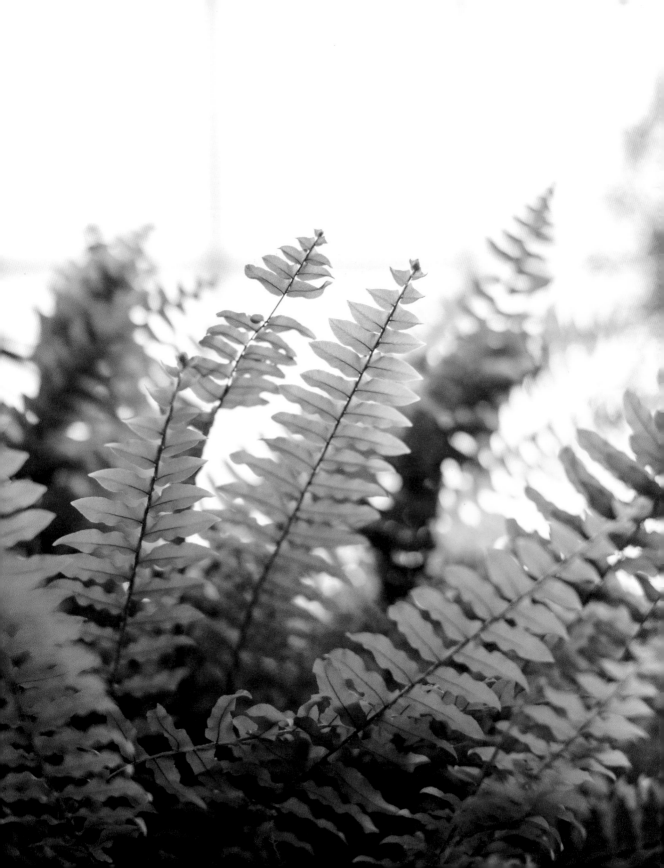

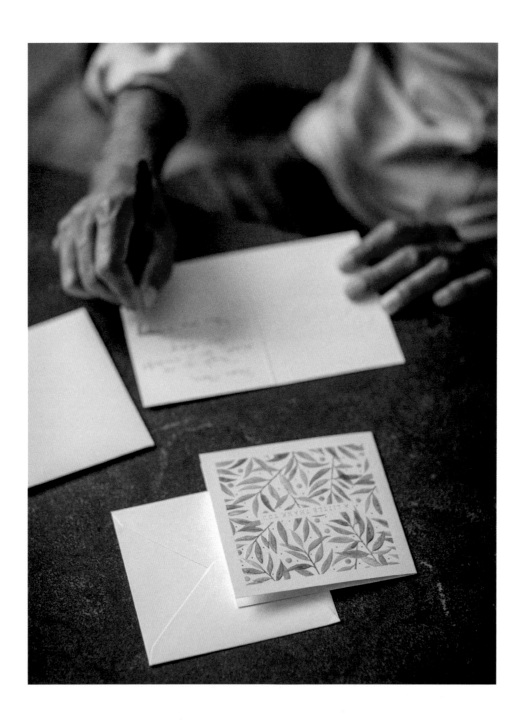

One Week of Kindness

Perform one act of kindness every day for a week. After you've completed each act of kindness, check in with yourself emotionally. How did it make you feel? If you find your Core Happiness is becoming noticeably stronger, keep performing acts of kindness.

Here are a few ideas to get you started:

- Go shopping for an elderly neighbour

- Cook a meal for someone outside your immediate family

- Send a text message in the evening, telling someone how much they mean to you

- Hold a door open for a stranger

- Tell your barista how wonderful the coffee is

- Buy a coffee for the person behind you in the queue

- Give your partner a foot massage

To really maximize the benefit, start a diary or journal and write down how many acts you have completed and how you felt afterwards.

Why not try to do this for at least one week every month?

Compassion-induced Meditation

A great method of giving yourself away to others, inside your own heart, is with a practice of Loving Kindness Meditation. This has been shown to reduce stress and increase happiness and empathy. It helps people become less focused on themselves, which can be associated with increased feelings of anxiety and depression, and helps them to feel closer to others, including strangers. You can practise for two minutes or twenty minutes, depending on the time you have available and your preference.

- Sit in a quiet space with your eyes closed. Take a deep belly-breath, in and out.

- Think of a person you feel close to. Imagine them standing next to you sending unconditional love to you. Feel their warmth and compassion flowing towards you.

- Focus on sending your own love back to that person. Remind yourself that this person is just like you – trying to do their best to have a happy and contented life.

- Now picture someone else you feel close to. Send warmth and love out to them. Some people find it helpful to say to themselves, 'May your life be filled with happiness, health and wellbeing.'

- When you feel ready, try the same technique with someone you are neutral about and perhaps do not know so well, such as a work colleague or a fellow parent from the school run. Trying this technique on someone you don't like is especially powerful.

- Finally, send love and compassion out to all people all over the globe. Say to yourself, 'Just as I wish to, may you live with ease, happiness and good health.'

- Finish with a deep belly-breath in and out.

- Take a moment to notice how you feel after this short meditation, in your body and in your mind.

- Open your eyes.

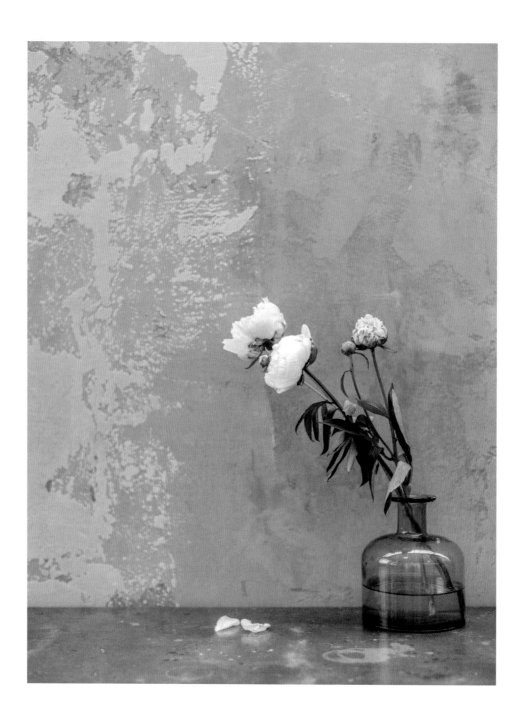

CONCLUSION

No one is an island. Humans survive and thrive in webs of connection. It's not by chance that the ultimate punishment in prisons is solitary confinement: being removed from social contact is a form of psychological torture. We can choose to experience the opposite of that hell when we give ourselves away. There's no greater feeling of freedom and lightness than when we sacrifice our own wants in service of others. It's as if all our selfish worries and obsessions melt away. This is life's most perfect irony: when we prioritize the happiness of others, it's ourselves who end up smiling.

A FINAL THOUGHT...

GET GOOD AT HAPPY

If there's one message I'd like you to take away from this book it's this: you can get good at happy. Happiness isn't some impossibly distant destination, or a state of mind reserved for the privileged. It's trainable and accessible to everyone. And, yes, that definitely means you.

Throughout these pages, I've broken down many scientifically proven ways you can strengthen your Core Happiness using simple practices that are mostly cheap or free. Many of them don't take a lot of time. I know there's an awful lot to choose from. Perhaps you feel slightly overwhelmed right now, and unsure where to begin. If so, my advice is to just start with one. That's all it takes. One intervention, that really speaks to you, for just a few minutes a day. After a week you'll be happier than you would've been otherwise. Then, choose another. And if you feel up to it, go for another.

If you practice happiness a little bit, you'll become a little bit happier. If you practice a lot, you'll become transformed. You'll find you have a brand-new relationship with yourself. You'll understand yourself in a way that's fresh and freeing and beautiful. You'll discover that much of your identity has been built *for* you, not by you; that you've been pushed into shape by our Want Brain culture, living in a cage that's been constructed for you. This book, I hope, has not only opened your eyes to this cage; it's given you the keys to the lock. It'll enable you to break out, a better, happier person than you ever thought possible.

Although I can give you the keys, I can't force you to put them in the lock. The only person who can do that is you. So, what are you waiting for?

It's time to start.

REFERENCES AND FURTHER READING

INTRODUCTION

https://pubmed.ncbi.nlm.nih.gov/17101814/
https://www.apa.org/pubs/journals/releases/psp805804.pdf
Daniel Nettle, *Happiness* (Oxford University Press, 2006 Kindle edition), pp. 67, 113

1. WRITE YOUR HAPPY ENDING

Daniel Nettle, *Happiness* (Oxford University Press, 2006 Kindle edition), Kindle location 1578
Jane McGonigal, *Reality is Broken: Why Games Make Us Better and How They Can Change the World* (Vintage, 2012), p. 31

2. ELIMINATE CHOICE

https://psycnet.apa.org/record/2000-16701-012
https://www.wsj.com/articles/BL-NB-309
https://web.archive.org/web/20070928231853/https://www.academie-amorim.com/us/laureat_2001/brochet.pdf
https://science.unctv.org/content/reportersblog/choices

3. TREAT YOURSELF WITH RESPECT

https://bmcpublichealth.biomedcentral.com/articles/10.1186/s12889-020-8183-1
https://self-compassion.org/wp-content/uploads/2015/04/Hiraoka_Meyer_etal SelfCompassionPredictsPTSD_JTS15.pdf
https://self-compassion.org/wp-content/uploads/2016/04/Shapira2010.pdf
https://self-compassion.org/wp-content/uploads/2020/06/Neff2020d.pdf
For more resources and further reading on self-compassion, please visit Dr Kristin Neff's website: https://self-compassion.org

4. MAKE TIME STAND STILL

https://journals.sagepub.com/doi/abs/10.1177/1948550615623842
https://www.pnas.org/content/pnas/114/32/8523.full.pdf

https://www.pewresearch.org/social-trends/2015/11/04/raising-kids-and-running-a-household-how-working-parents-share-the-load

https://www.hbs.edu/ris/Publication%20Files/Time,%20Money,%20and%20Subjective%20Well-Being_cb363d54-6410-4049-9cf5-9d7b3bc94bcb.pdf

https://pubmed.ncbi.nlm.nih.gov/16698116

Gary Rogowski, *Handmade: Creative Focus in the Age of Destruction* (Linden Publishing, 2017)

Steven Kotler, *The Art of Impossible* (HarperWave, 2021)

5. SEEK OUT FRICTION

Edith Eger, *The Choice* (Rider, 2018) and *The Gift: Twelve Lessons to Save Your Life* (Rider, 2020)

John McAvoy, *Redemption: From Iron Bars to Iron Man* (Pitch, 2019)

https://www.bbc.co.uk/sport/54601706

https://drchatterjee.com/if-this-man-can-turn-his-life-around-so-can-you/

6. TALK TO STRANGERS

https://www.adultdevelopmentstudy.org

Paul A. M. van Lange and Simon Columbus, 'Vitamin S: Why is Social Contact, Even with Strangers, so Important to Well-Being?', *Current Directions in Psychological Science* (in press)

https://psycnet.apa.org/record/2014-28833-001?doi=1

https://www.bbc.co.uk/news/world-48459940

https://www.ncbi.nlm.nih.gov/pmc/articles/PMC2944762/

https://journals.sagepub.com/doi/abs/10.1177/1948550613502990

https://doi.org/10.1007/s12144-018-9886-7

https://copeify.com/mentalhealth/2020/11/29/the-surprising-benefits-of-talking-to-strangers

7. TREAT YOUR PHONE LIKE A PERSON

https://www.journals.uchicago.edu/doi/abs/10.1086/691462

https://journals.sagepub.com/doi/full/10.1177/0265407518769387

https://www.sciencedirect.com/science/article/abs/pii/S0747563218304643

https://www.bbfc.co.uk/about-us/news/children-see-pornography-as-young-as-seven-new-report-finds

https://www.visualcapitalist.com/the-50-most-visited-websites-in-the-world/

https://journals.lww.com/jrnldbp/Abstract/2014/04000/Pornography_and_Sexual_Experiences_Among_High.3.aspx

8. HAVE MASKLESS CONVERSATIONS

https://thehill.com/changing-america/well-being/mental-health/542186-new-stanford-study-says-zoom-calls-trigger-our

https://www.ncbi.nlm.nih.gov/pmc/articles/PMC2944762/

https://eprints.mdx.ac.uk/10847/1/Lenton_Bruder_Slabu_Sedikides_PhenomenologyAuthenticity_2012.pdf

https://journals.sagepub.com/doi/full/10.1037/gpr0000162

Carl Rogers and Peter Kramer, *On Becoming a Person: A Therapist's View of Psychotherapy* (Robinson, 1977)

9. GO ON HOLIDAY EVERY DAY

https://www.ncbi.nlm.nih.gov/pmc/articles/PMC6137615/

https://www.ncbi.nlm.nih.gov/pmc/articles/PMC7287297/

https://pubmed.ncbi.nlm.nih.gov/24107199/

https://www.ncbi.nlm.nih.gov/pmc/articles/PMC3772979/

10. GIVE YOURSELF AWAY

https://pubmed.ncbi.nlm.nih.gov/18356530/

https://www.tandfonline.com/doi/abs/10.1080/07347324.2011.538320

https://www.ncbi.nlm.nih.gov/pmc/articles/PMC4851591/

https://pubmed.ncbi.nlm.nih.gov/24853935/

https://www.apa.org/pubs/journals/releases/hea-31-1-87.pdf

https://journals.sagepub.com/doi/abs/10.1177/0956797612442551

https://pubmed.ncbi.nlm.nih.gov/29702043/

Oliver Scott Curry *et al.*, 'Happy to help? A systematic review and meta-analysis of the effects of performing acts of kindness on the well-being of the actor', *Journal of Experimental Social Psychology*, Vol. 76, 2018, 320–29

https://authors.library.caltech.edu/66351/

INDEX

Abel, Julian 251
addiction 73–4, 77
    pornography 179–80
albums 56, 59
alignment 16, 17
    daily holidays 208–236
    and flow 102
    and friction 110–31
    give yourself away 238–61
    journalling 228
    judging others 122
    maskless conversations
        184–207
    and phones 156–83
    and religion 250
    and self-talk 67
    treat yourself with respect
        66–85
    why it matters 40–42
    write your happy ending
        24–45
Alter, Adam 161
Amazon 168
anandamide 102
Auschwitz 114
authenticity 194–5, 196

Bailenson, Jeremy 192
breathwork 219, 230
Buddhism 215

Carver, Courtney 56
CDs 34, 56
choice 47–8, 61
    affecting health 52–5
    false versus meaningful
        choices 50–51
    ways to eliminate 56–9

Columbus, Simon 135
compassion *see* self-
        compassion
compassion-induced
        meditation 258–9
competitiveness 28, 30, 63,
        74, 85
contentment 16, 17
    and choice 50
    daily holidays 208–236
    and flow 102
    and friction 110–31
    give yourself away 238–61
    judging others 122
    and phones 156–83
    and religion 249–50
    and self-talk 67
    and time 86–108
    control 16, 17
    and choice 46–61
    daily holidays 208–236
    and flow 102
    and friction 110–31
    give yourself away 238–61
    judging others 122
    maskless conversations
        184–207
    and phones 156–83
    and religion 249
    and self-talk 67
    talking to strangers
        132–54
    and time 86–108
    treat yourself with respect
        66–85
convenience 140–41
Core Happiness 16–17, 263
    and choice 50–51

and flow 102
    judging others 122–3
    and religion 249–50
    and self-talk 67
    and time 91
    see also alignment;
        contentment; control
creativity 104
criticism, dealing with 128–9
Csikszentmihalyi, Mihaly 102

daily holidays 208–210, 214,
        226–7, 236
    benefits 214
    breathwork 230
    and health 224–5
    journalling 228
    meditation 233
    movement 215–16
    routine to ritual 234–5
    sitting stillness 219–23
    solitude 212–13
dopamine 102
dreams 26–8
Dunn, Elizabeth 239
Durga Puja 242

Eger, Edith 114, 115
empathy 204–5
endorphins 102
Epley, Nicholas 135–6, 137,
        140, 245

film shortlist 58
flow 102–7, 108
    and gratitude 245
forgiveness 244
freedom 48

ACKNOWLEDGEMENTS

Books and podcasts can change the world. I truly believe that. So much of the information we consume these days is edited down and over-simplified. As a society, what we need is more nuance, perspective and compassion. This is exactly what long-form podcasts and books, like this one, give us. They allow us to deepen our understanding of who we really are.

My own life has been enhanced immeasurably by having weekly in-depth conversations on my podcast, 'Feel Better, Live More'. They have helped me refine and develop my thinking on a whole variety of different subjects, and many of the insights I have had as a consequence have ended up in the book that you now hold in your hands.

My hope is that this book provides value not just the first time you read it but for many years to come. I believe that the ideas it contains will take on a different meaning as you progress through life, and that you'll feel called to revisit them regularly.

Writing a manuscript and then transforming black and white words into a beautifully designed book is a team effort. I am grateful to have many people in my personal and professional life who believe in what I do and are dedicated to helping me spread my message as far and wide as possible.

To Vidhaata – you walk alongside me in everything that I do. You help me get to know myself better and I truly appreciate everything you do for me and our beautiful family. Thank you for your honesty, integrity, support and love. Thank you for being you.

To Jainam and Anoushka – spending time with you both is my very favourite Happiness Habit. You both inspire me to become a better person and have taught me the true meaning of success. Thank you both for the love, presence and joy you bring into my life.

To my family and friends – you know who you are – thank you for the unconditional support and always having my back.

Thank you to my team who work tirelessly to help me spread my message – Clare, Gareth, Sarah, Steph, Jeremy and Sophie – I appreciate every single one of you.

Special thanks to Will Storr, Will Francis and Sophie Laurimore.

Helen Hall – exchanging voice messages back and forth with you has helped me work through many of the ideas within this book. You are a special human being and I am lucky to know you.

Pippa Grange and Julia Samuel – thank you both for taking the time to read the manuscript and provide such valuable feedback. You are both special people doing incredible work.

My team at Penguin Life – my fifth book in five years . . . how on earth did that happen?! You are an incredible team and it has been a pleasure to work with you all again. Thank you for believing in me and my mission.

Christopher Terry – your photography is exquisite and has enhanced this book immeasurably.

I would like to extend a special thanks to Peter Crone, Gabor Mate, John McAvoy, Edith Eger, Greg McKeown, David Bradford, Carole Robin and Laurie Santos for the life-enhancing conversations on my 'Feel Better, Live More' podcast.

Thank you to every single one of my patients. You have taught me much more than I have taught you.

And, lastly, I would like to thank you, my reader, for picking up this book. Time is a valuable resource – the most precious one we have. Thank you for giving me some of yours. I appreciate it.

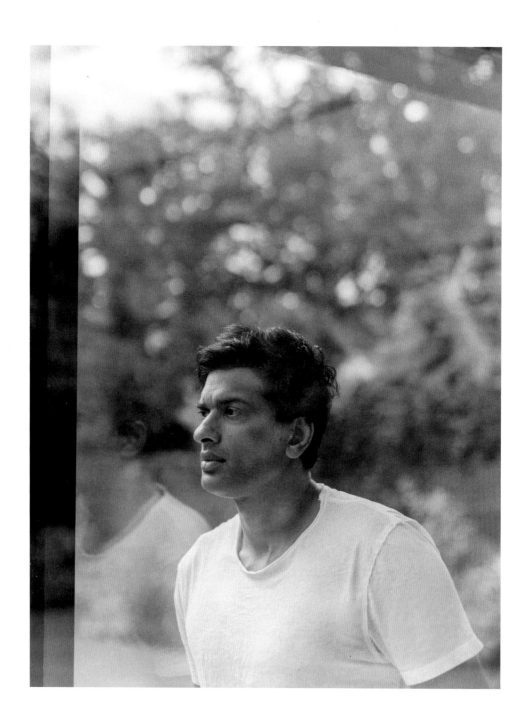